A beautiful photo book of North American birds

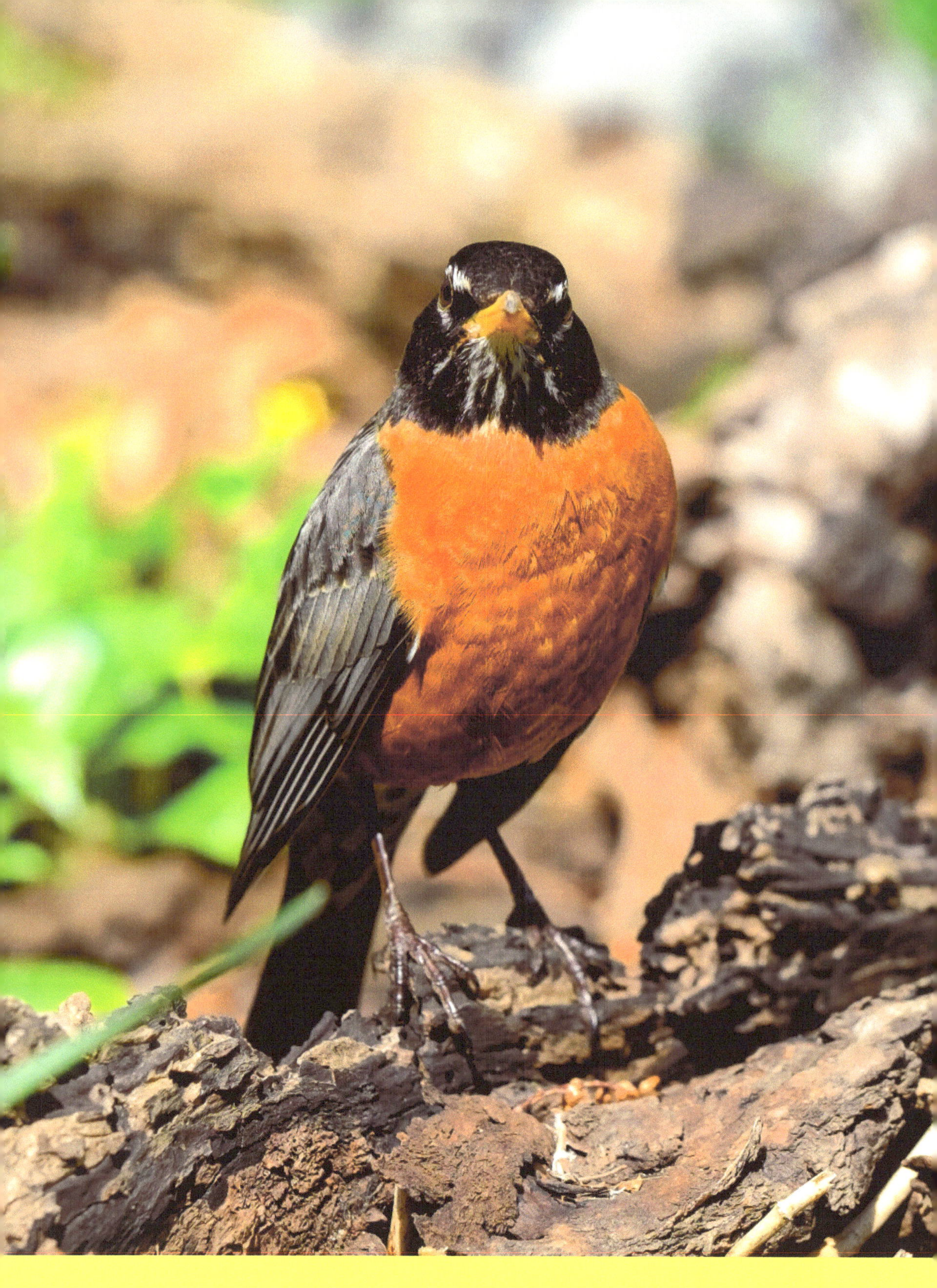

American Robin

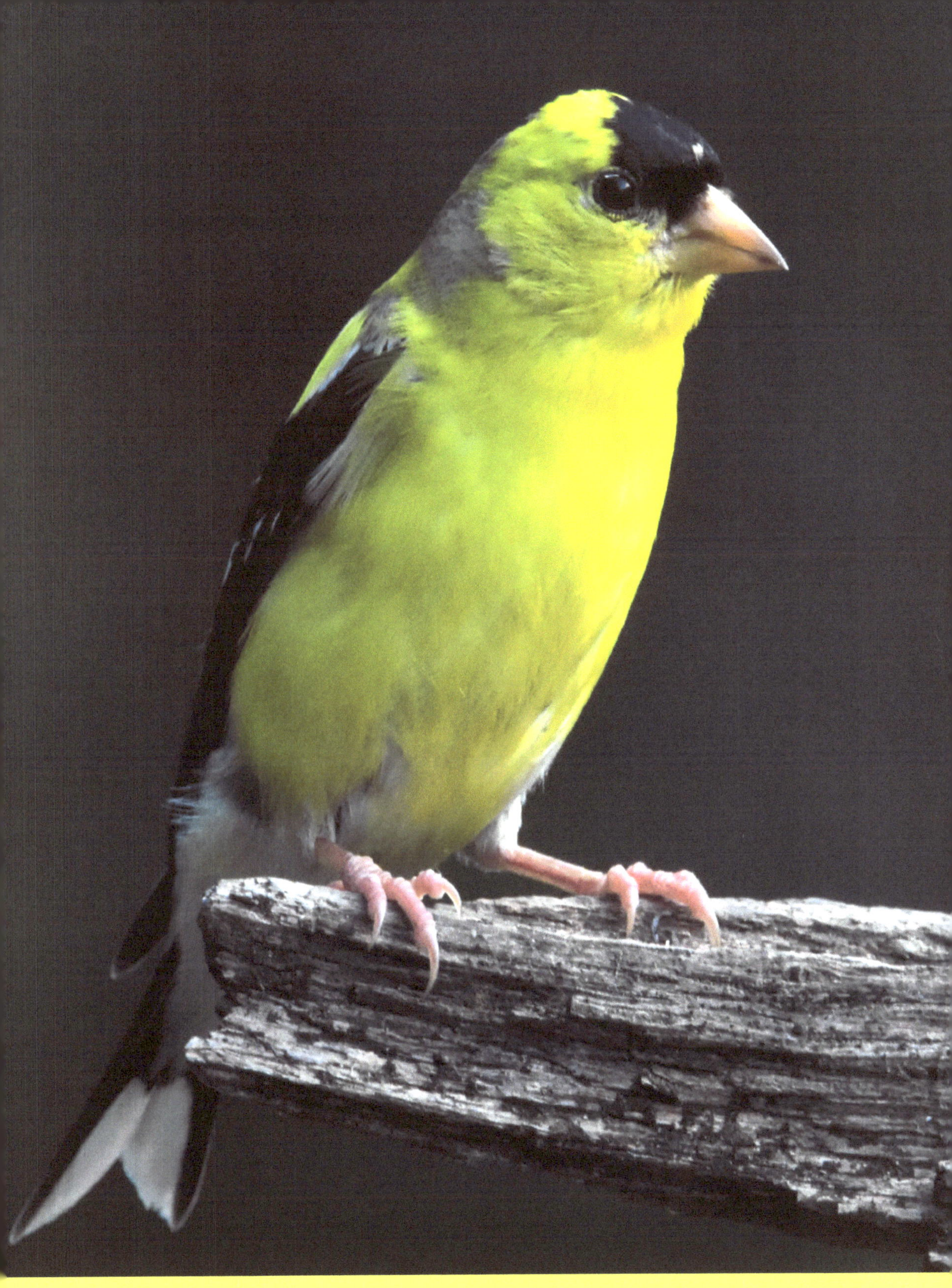

American Goldfinch

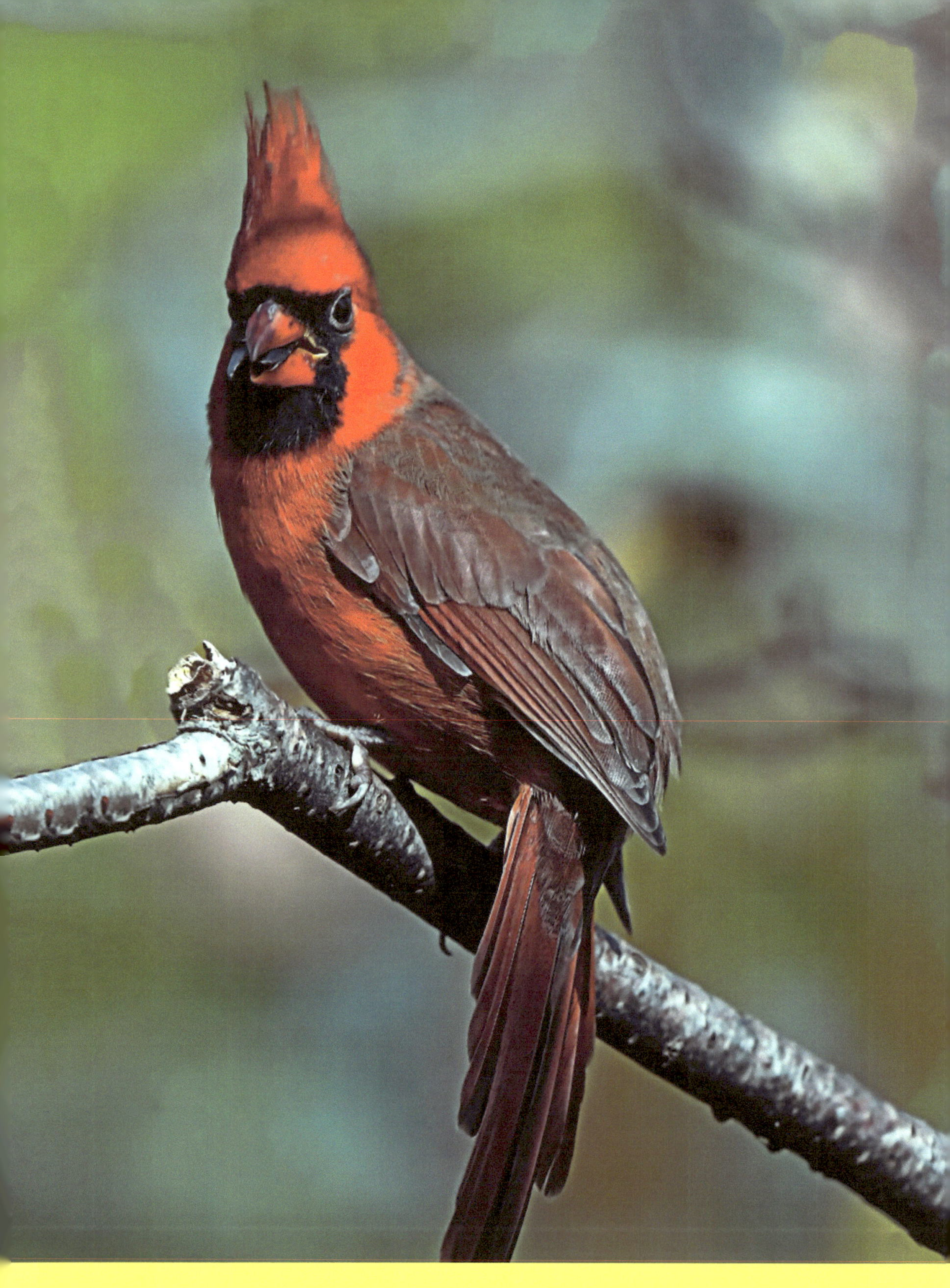

Northern Cardinal

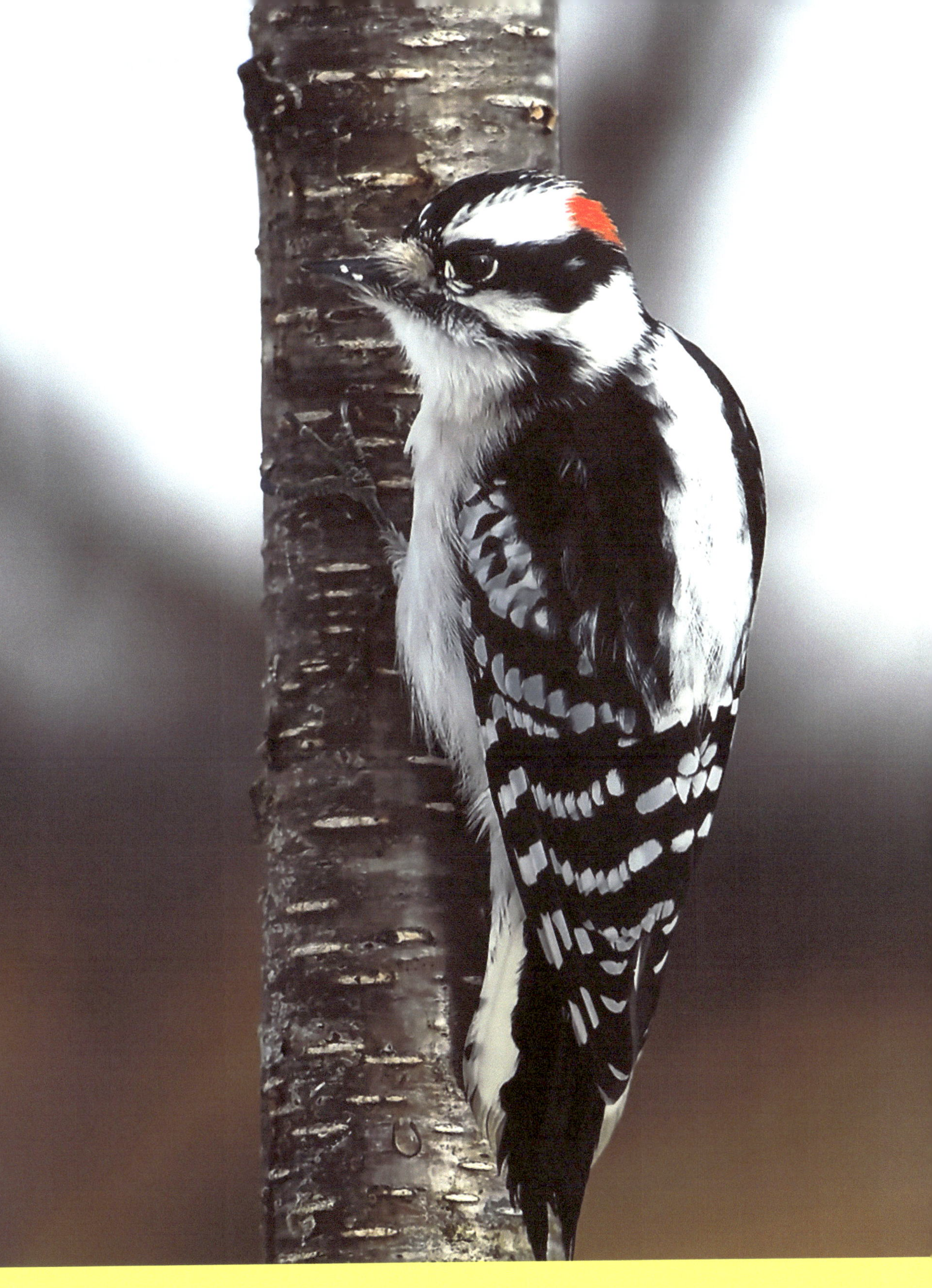

Downy Woodpecker

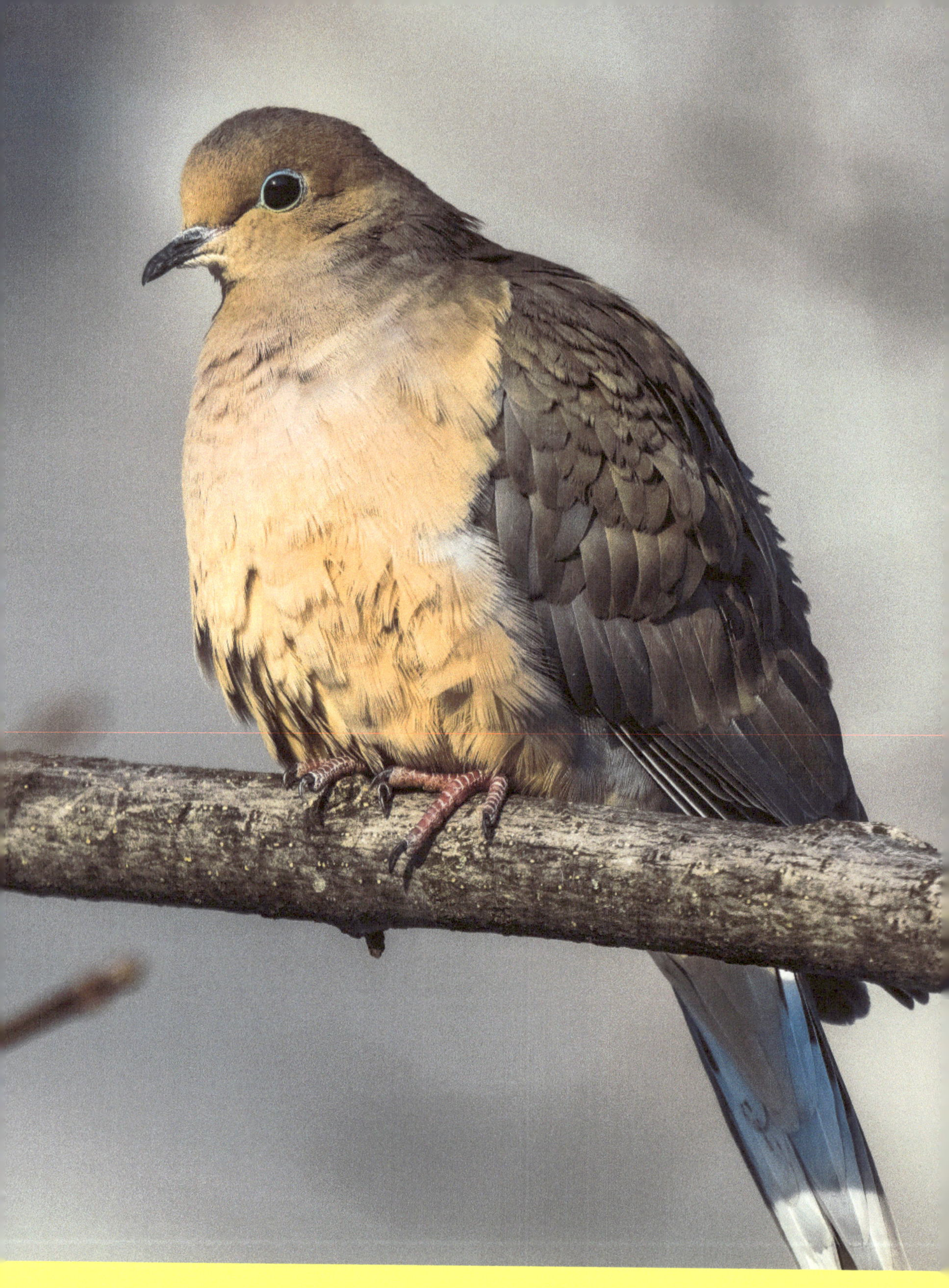

Mourning Dove

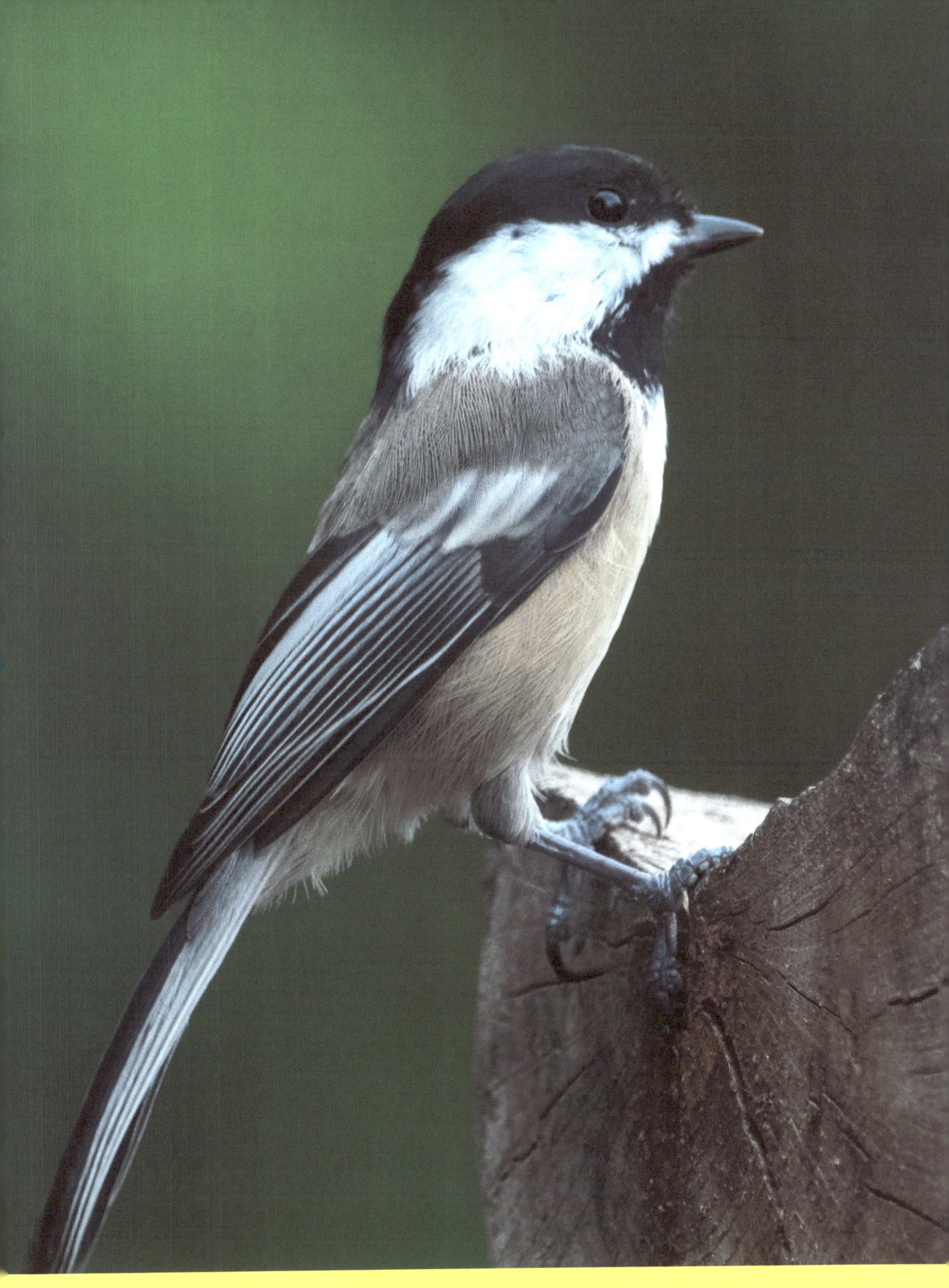

Black-capped Chickadee

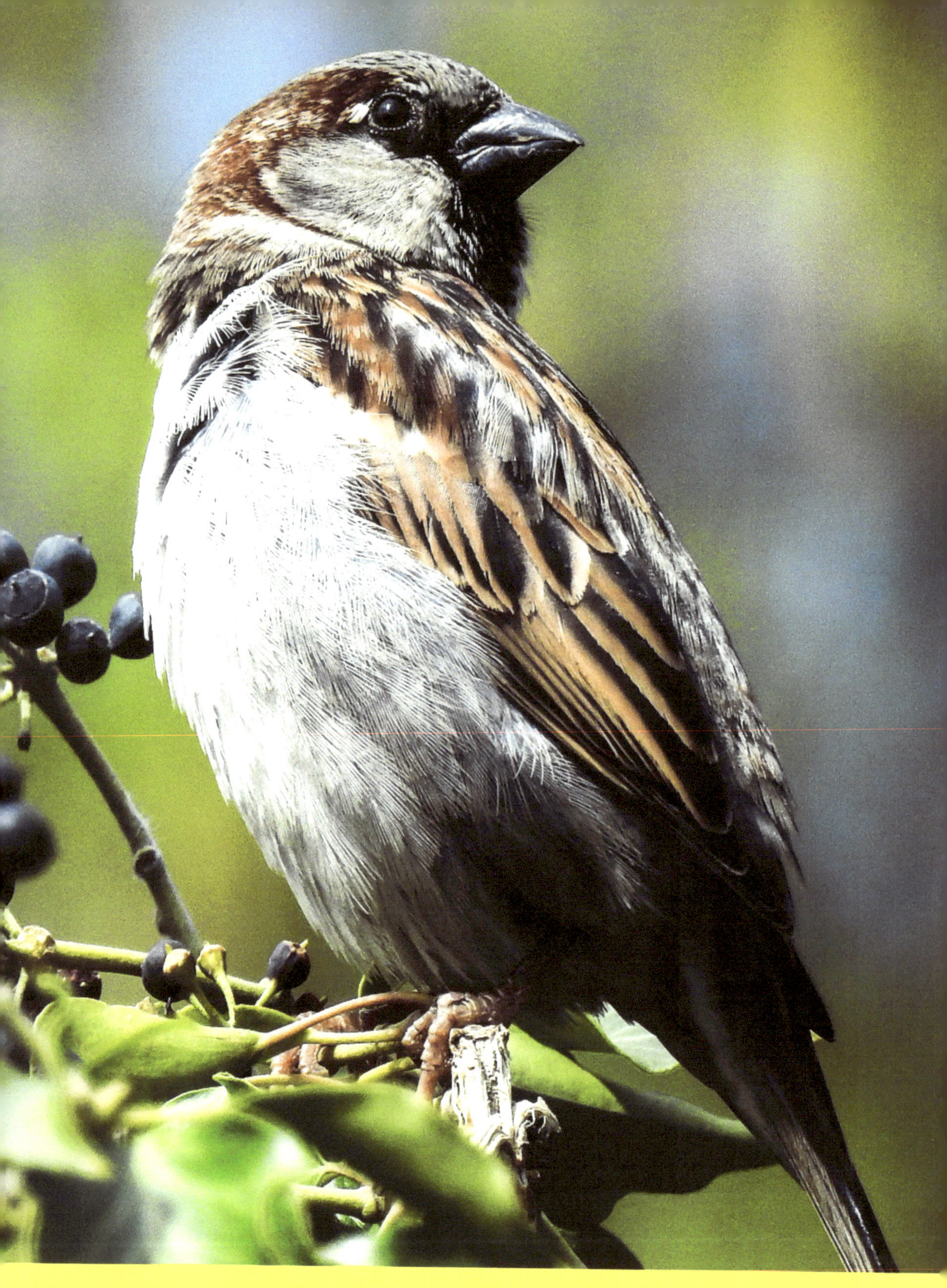

House Sparrow

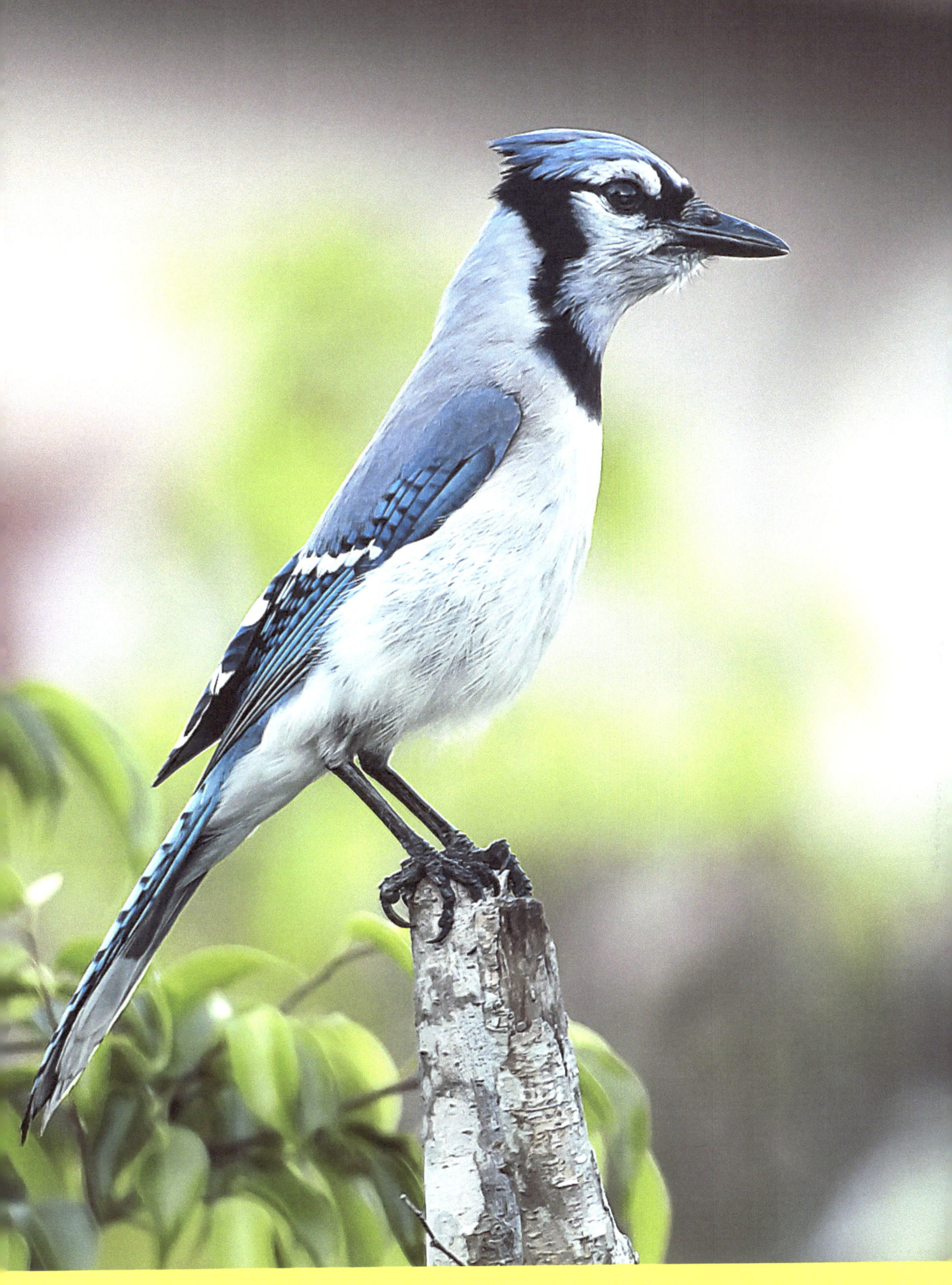

Blue Jay

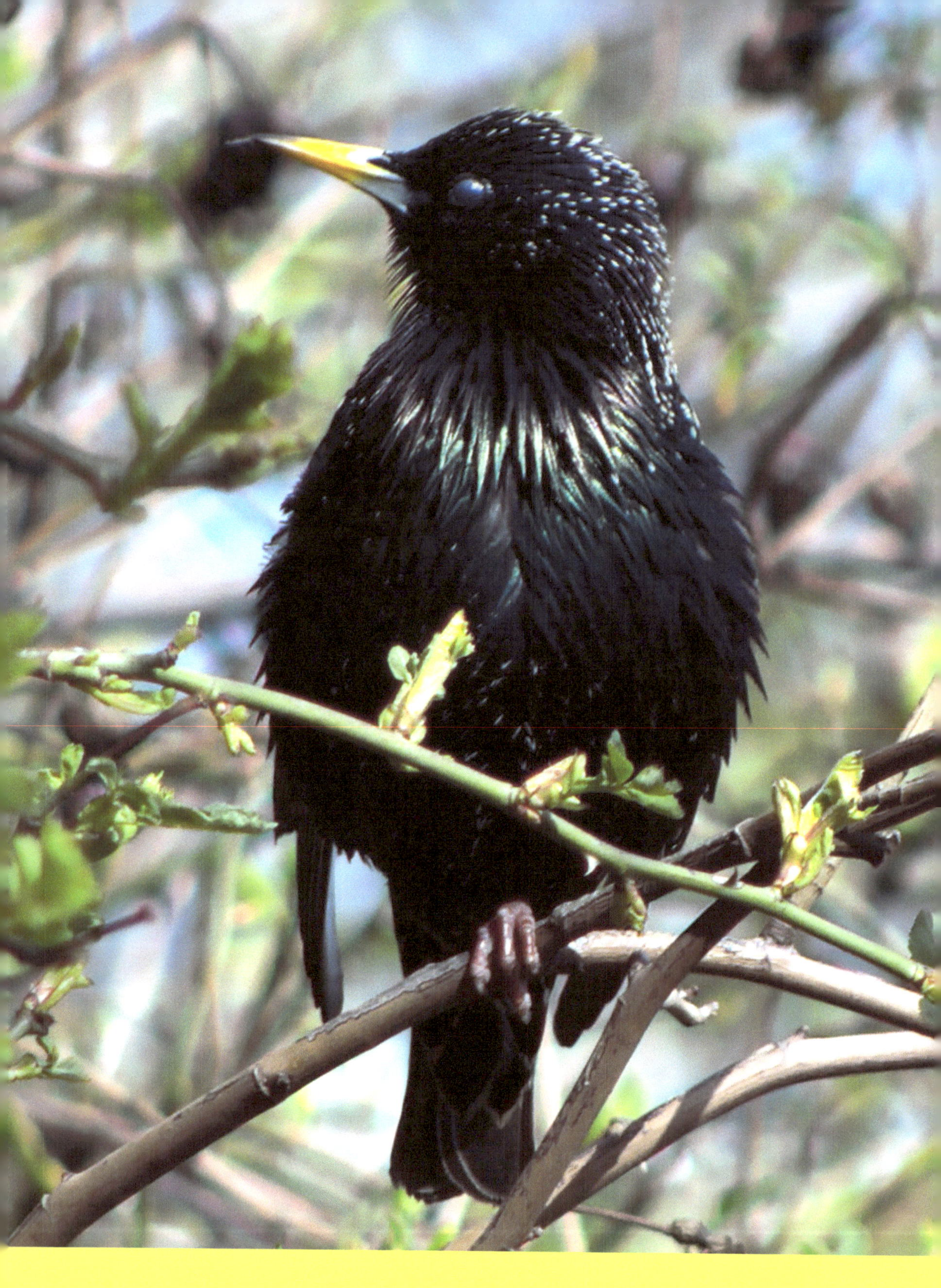

Common Starling

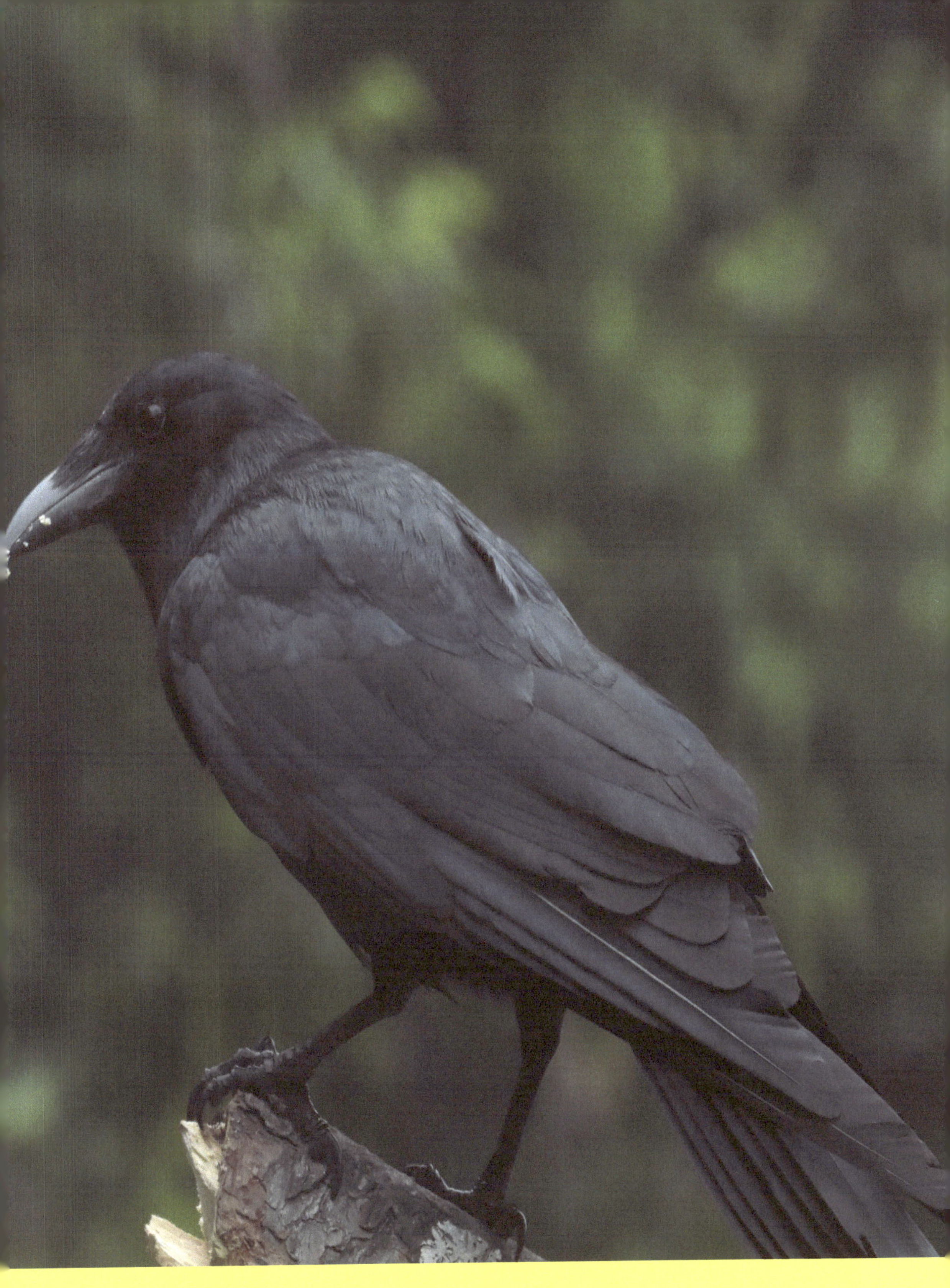

American Crow

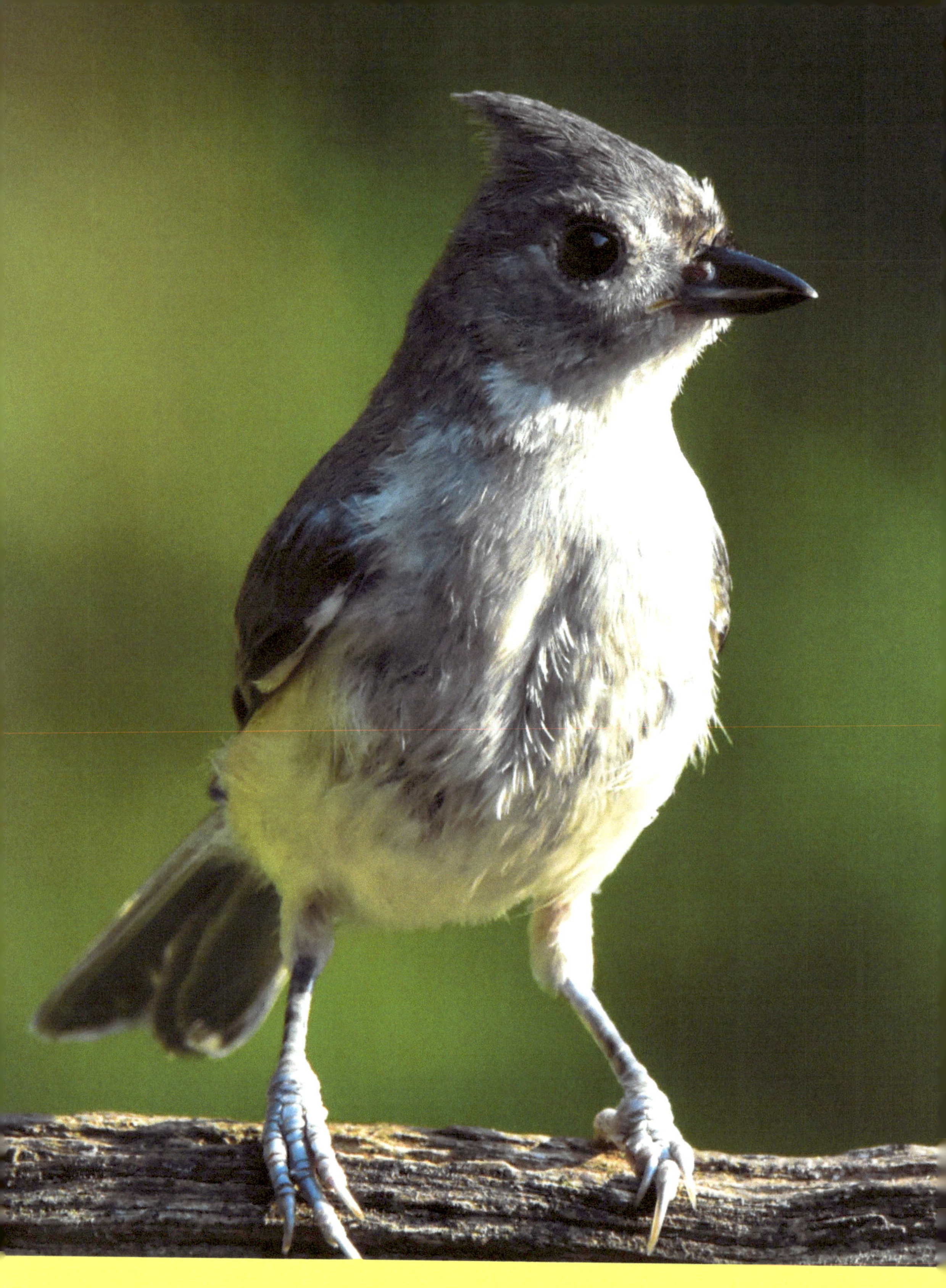

Tufted Titmouse

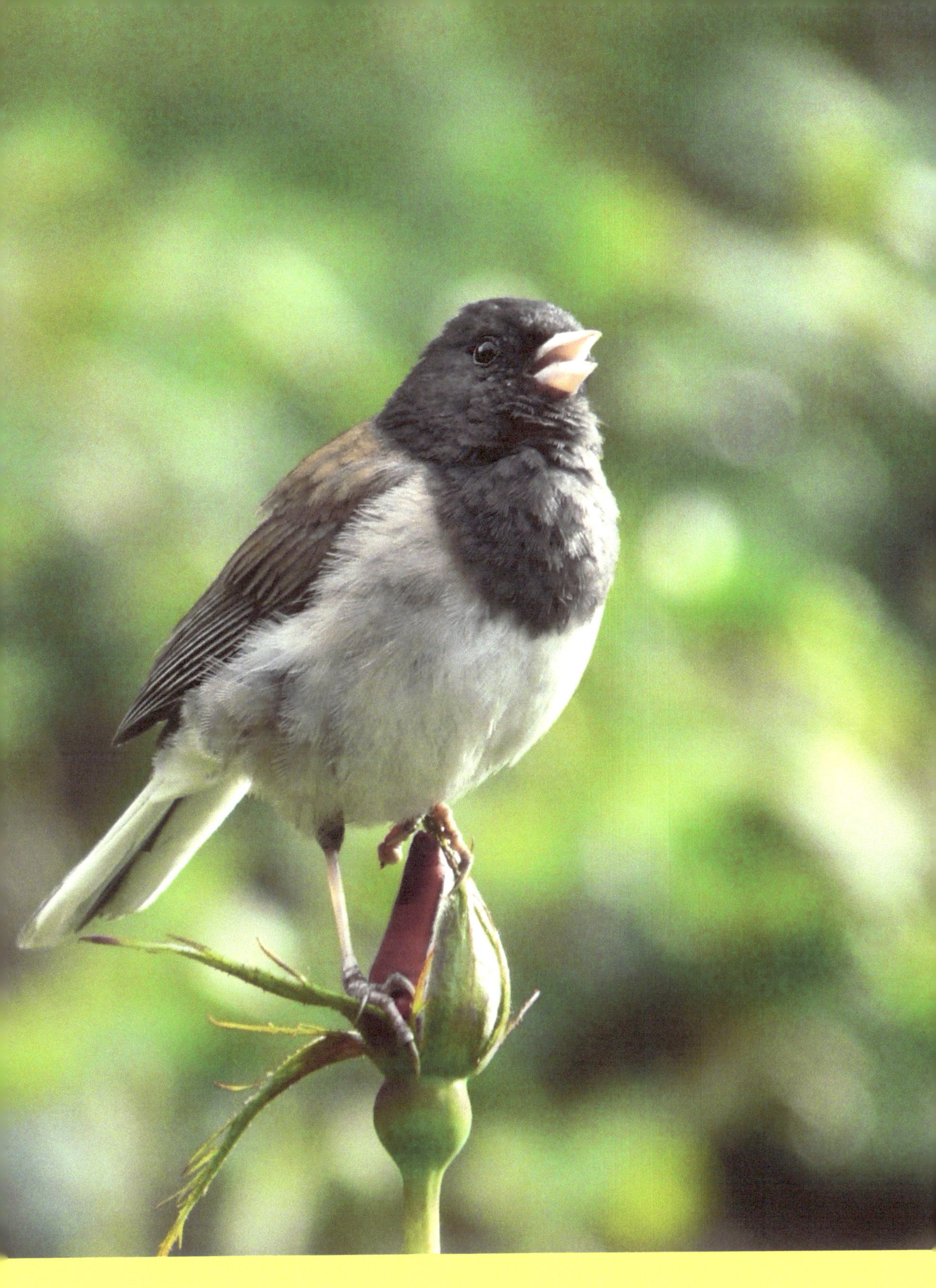

Dark-eyed Junco

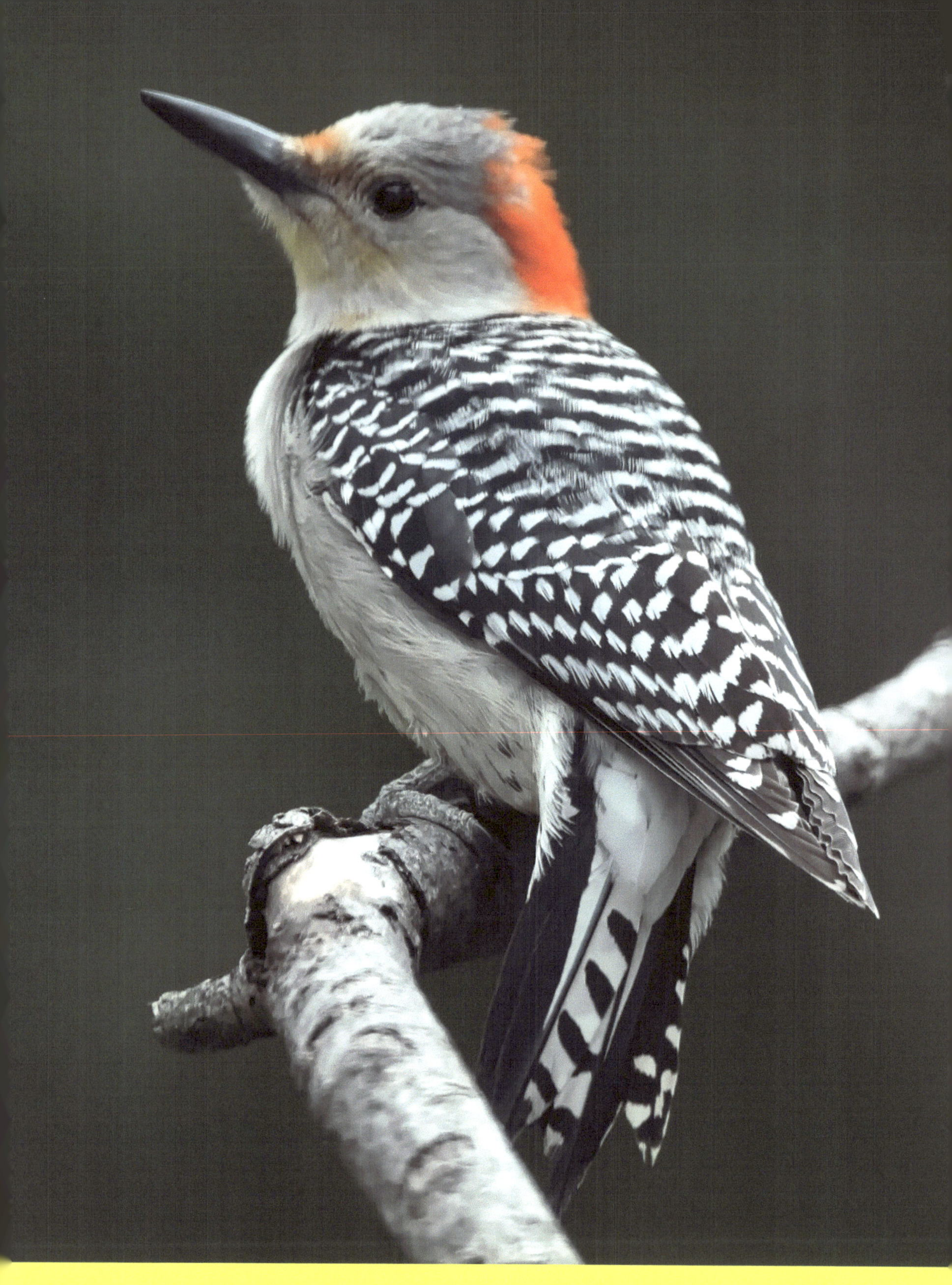

Red-bellied Woodpecker

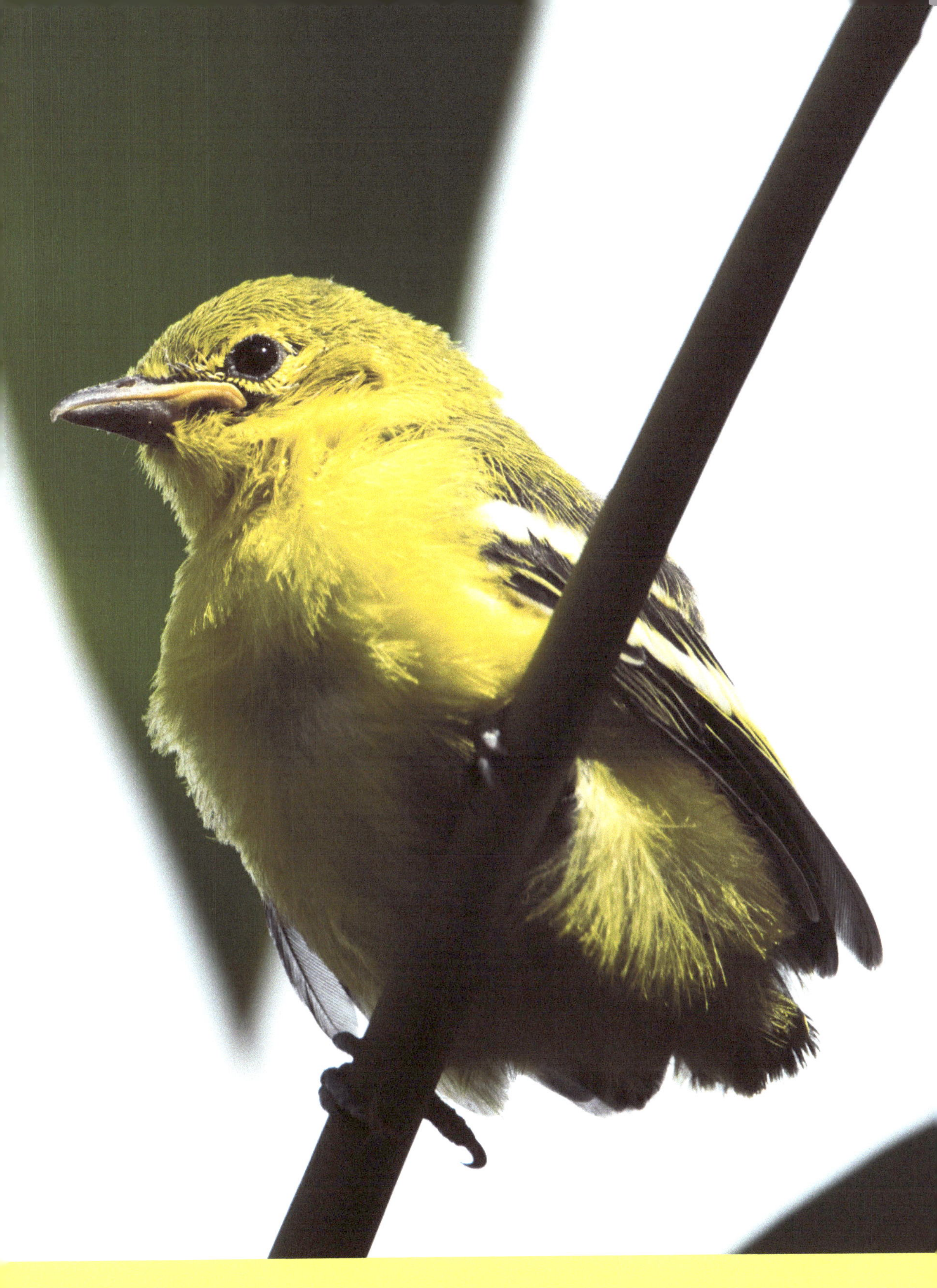

Yellow Rumped Warbler

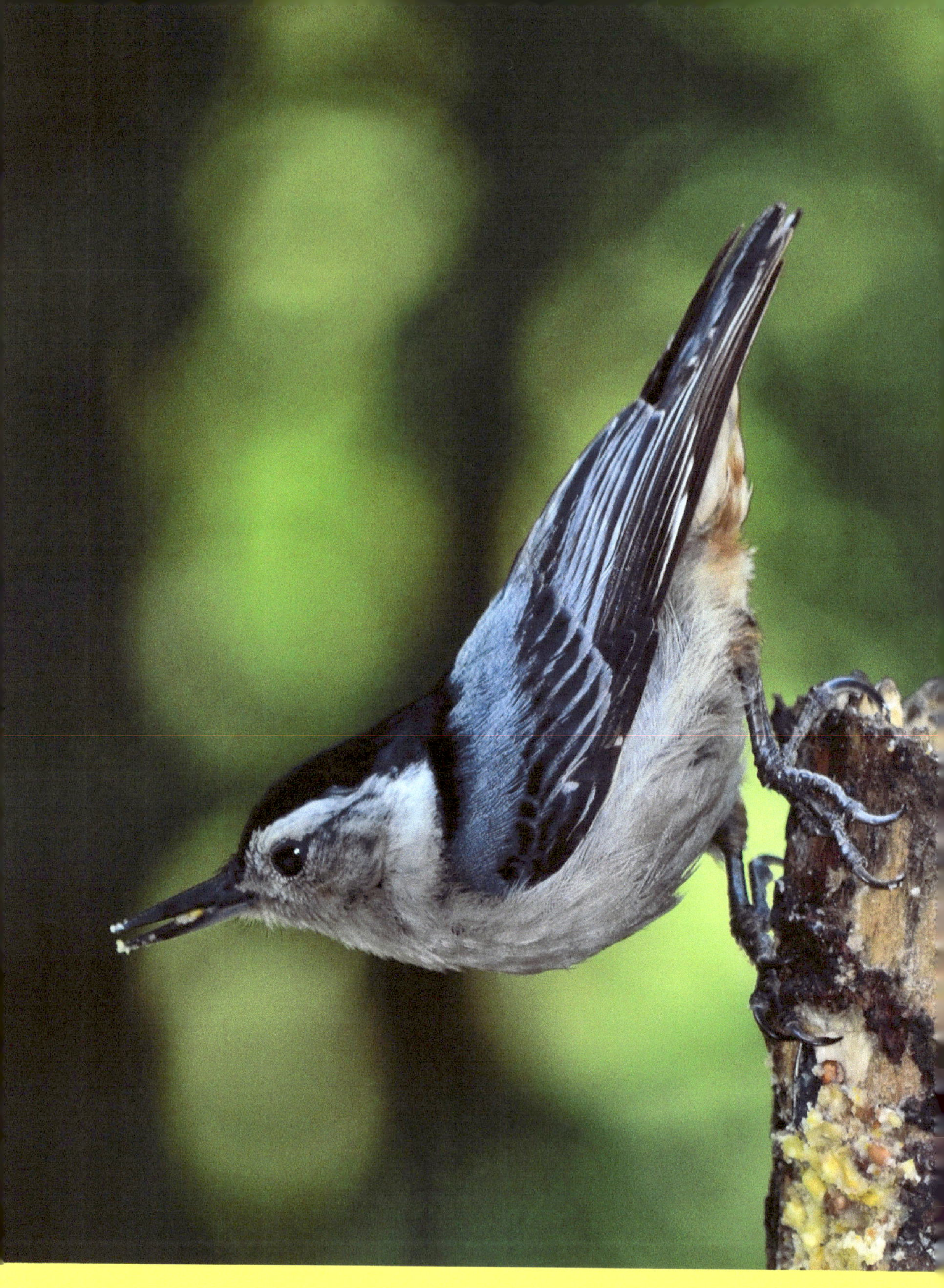

Nuthatch

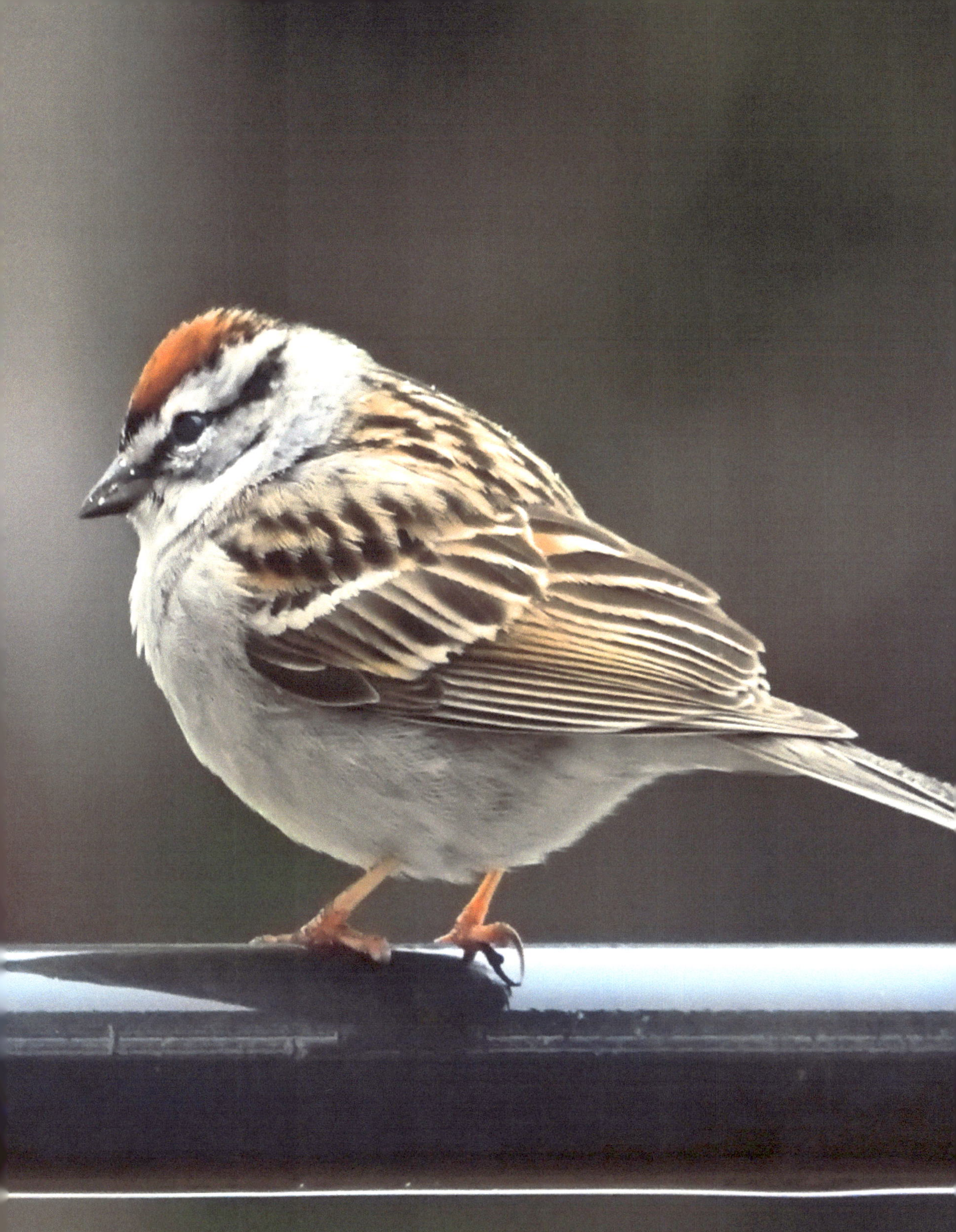

Chipping Sparrow

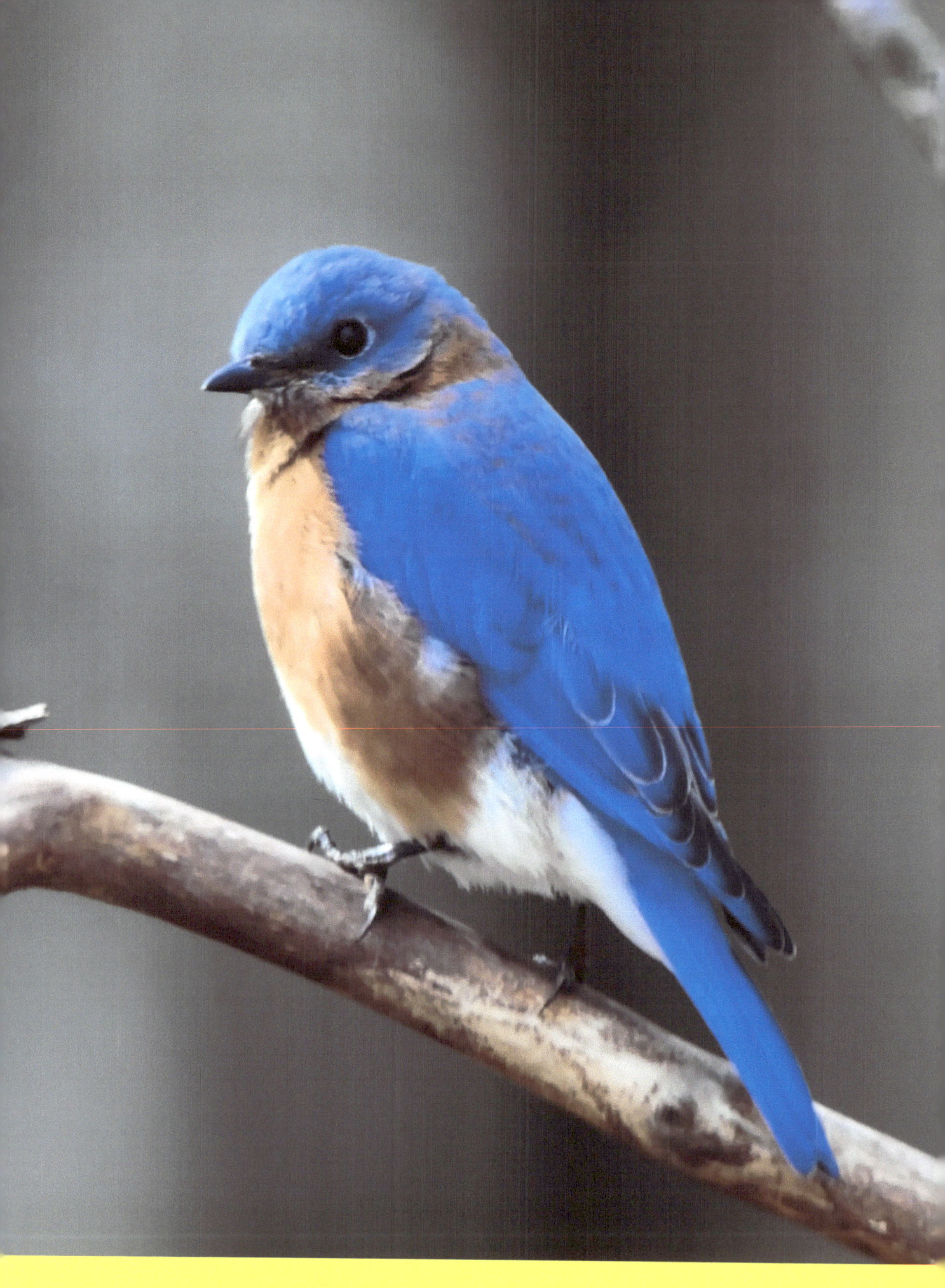

Eastern Bluebird

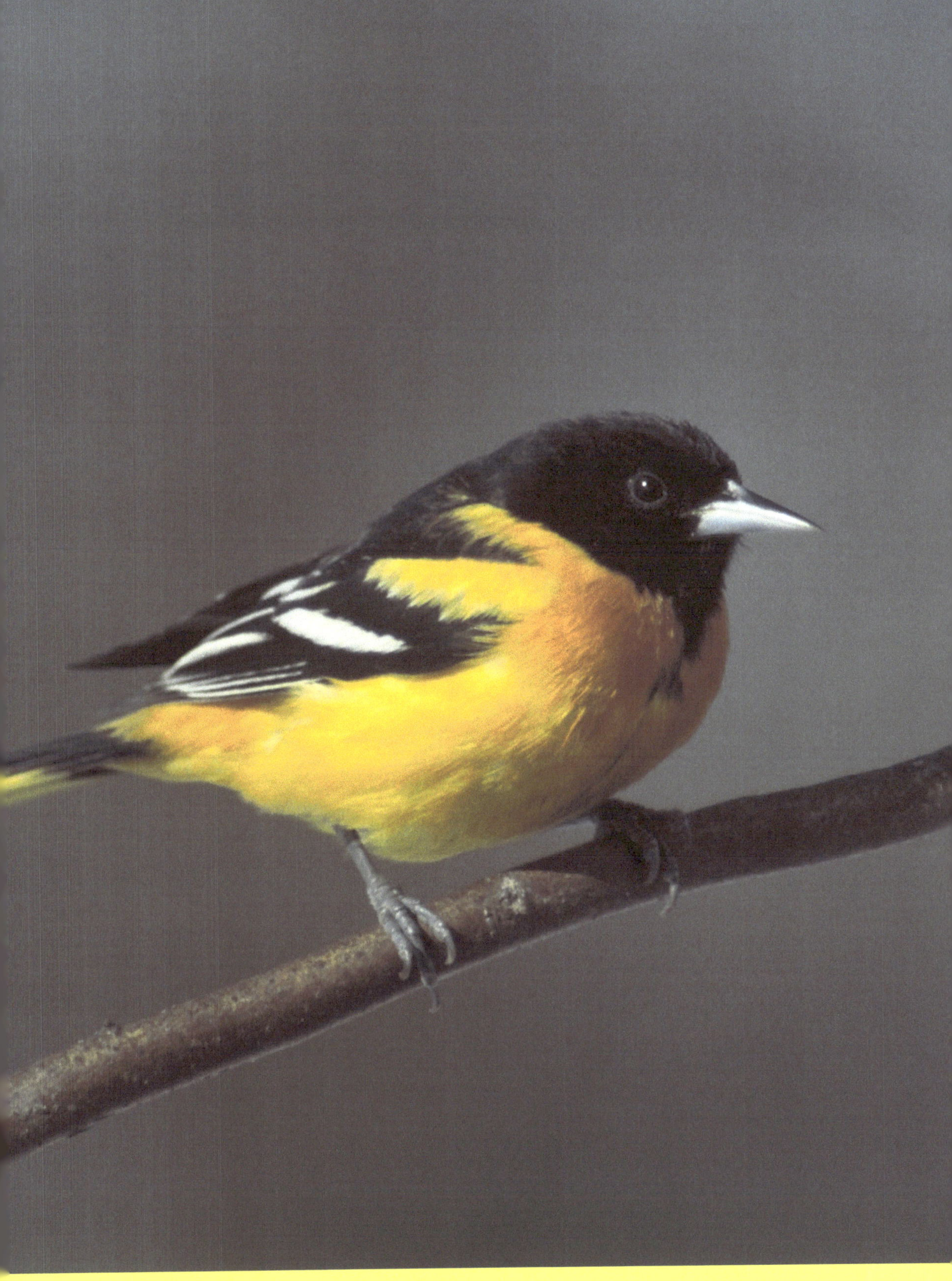

Baltimore Oriole

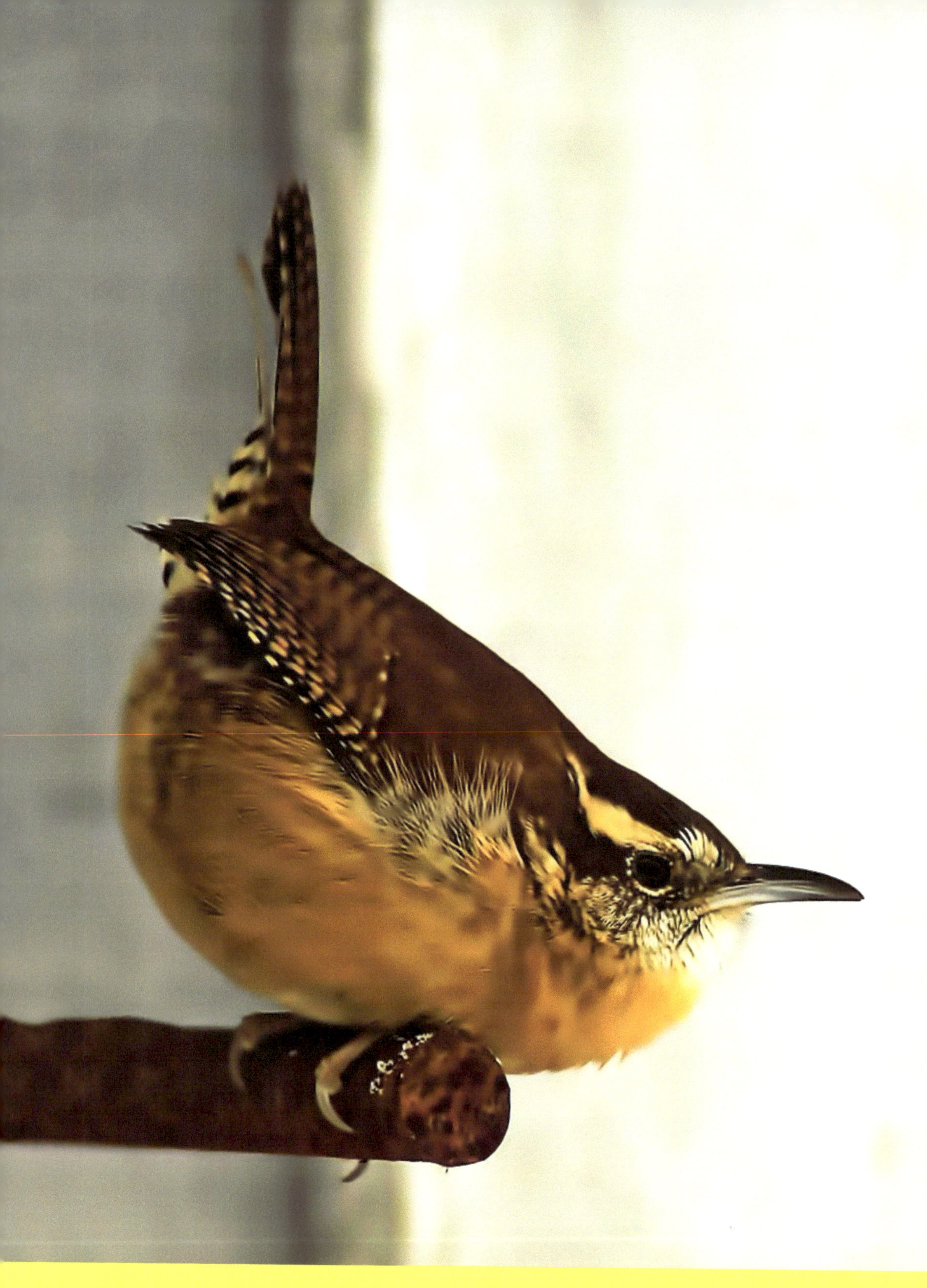

Carolina Wren

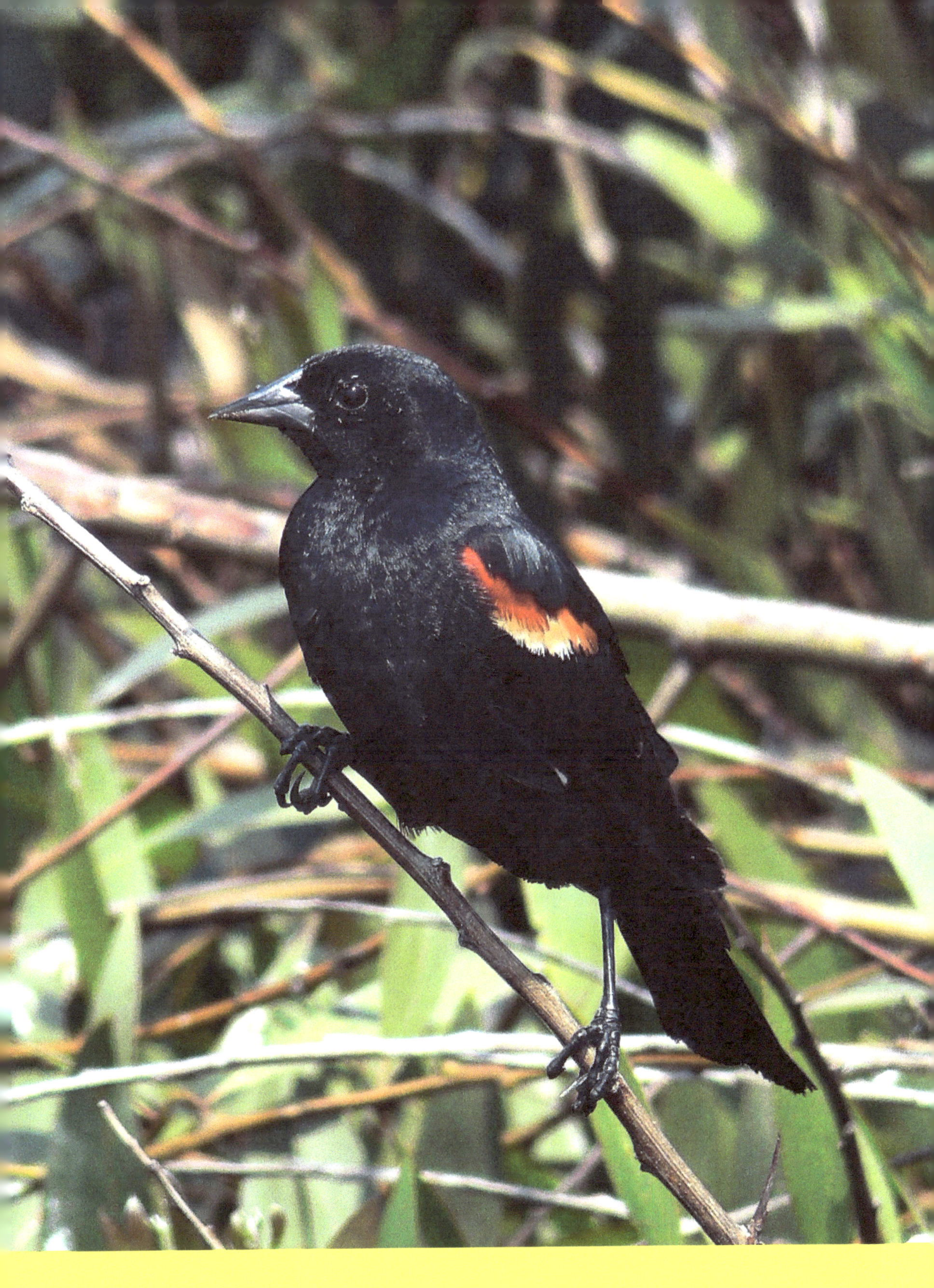

Red-winged Blackbird

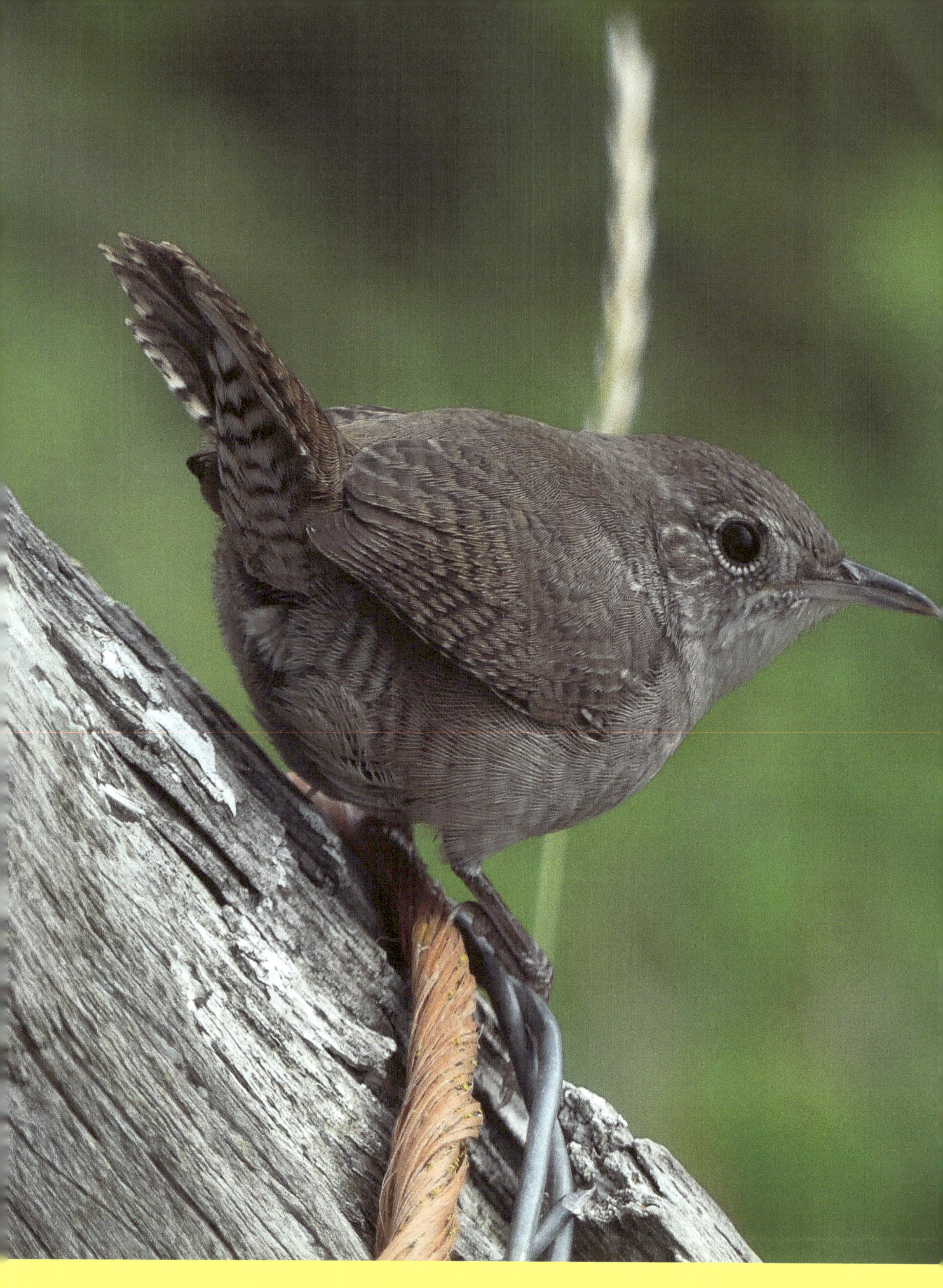

House Wren

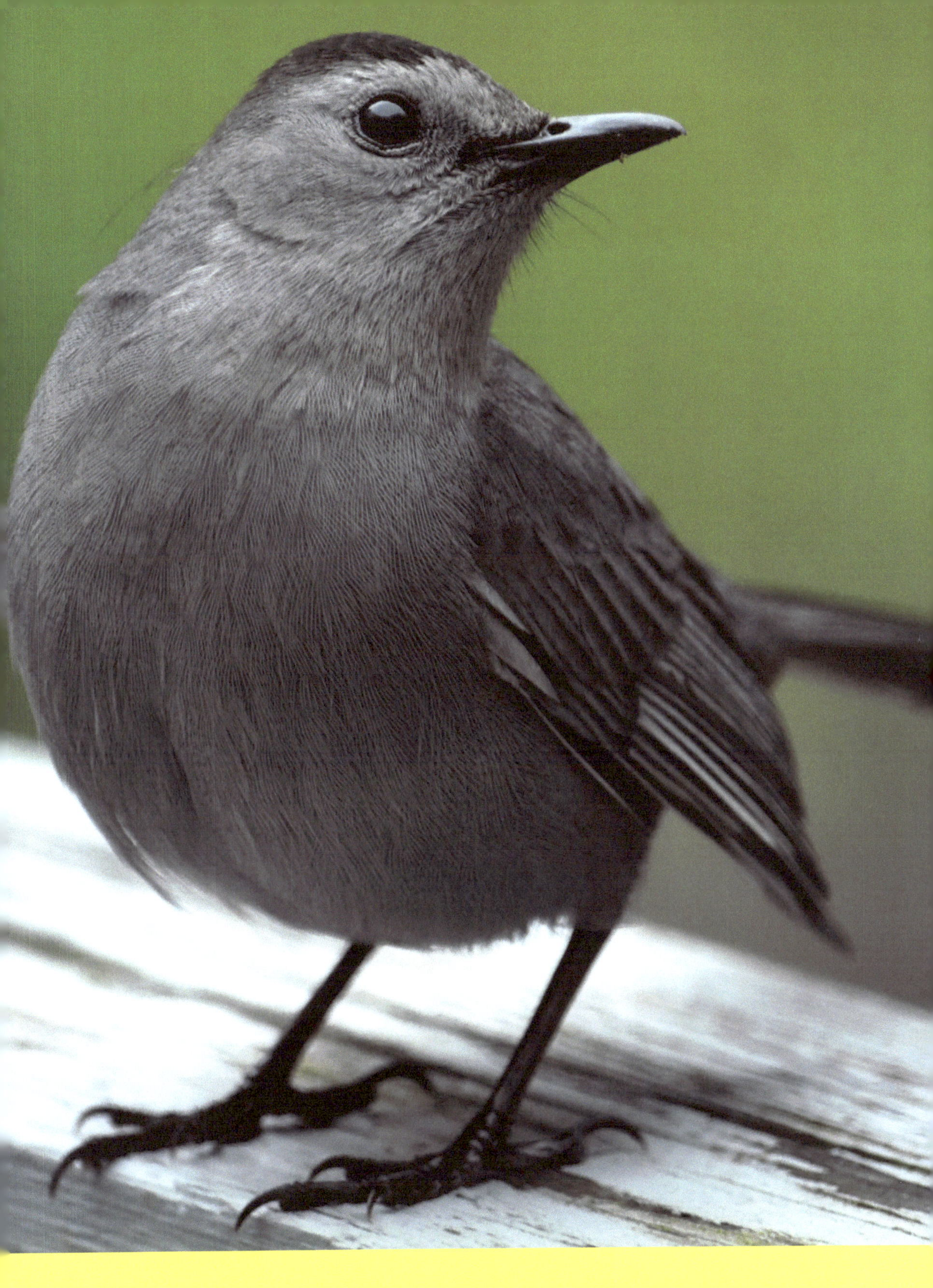

Gray catbird

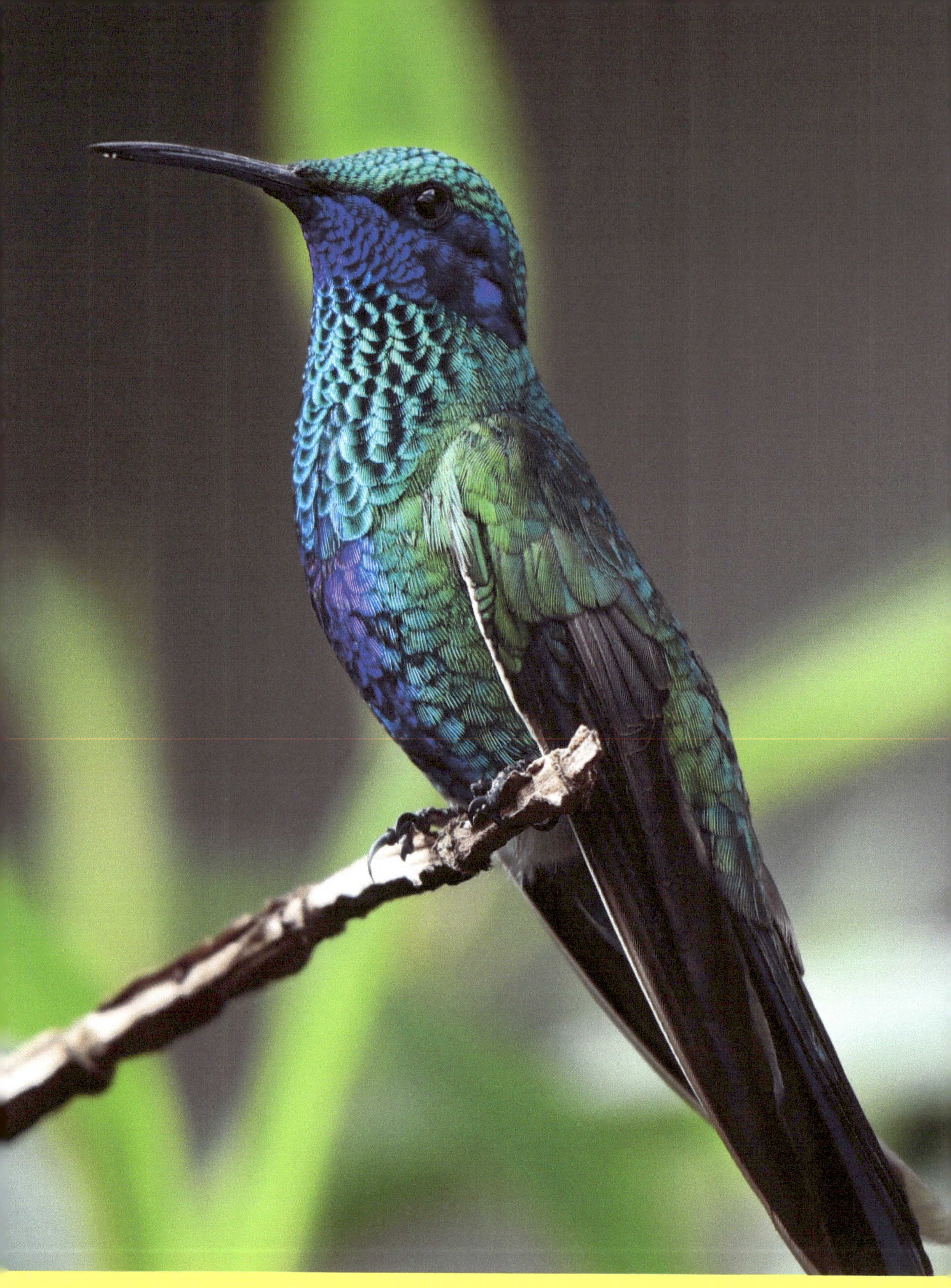

Hummingbird

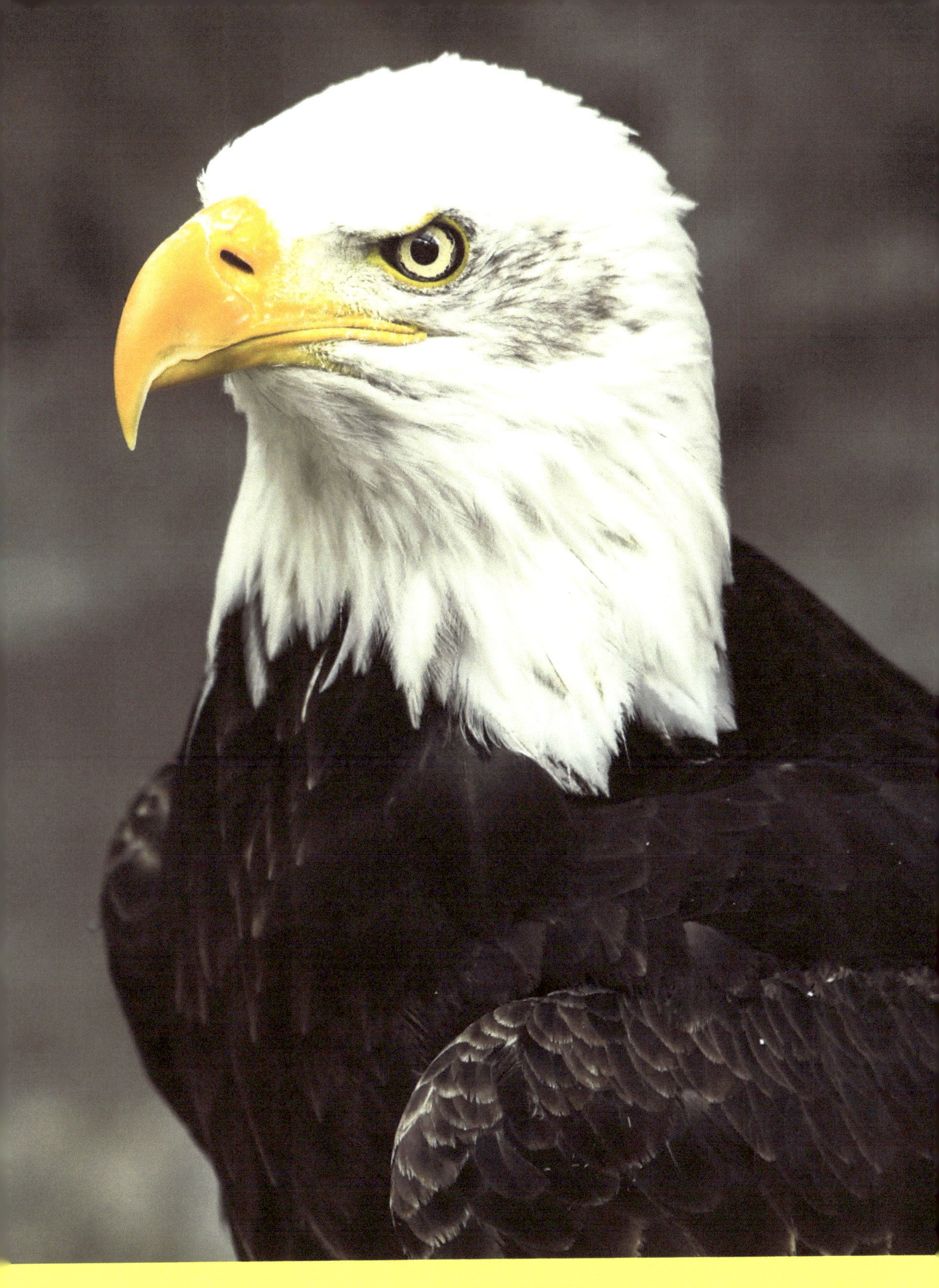

Bald Eagle

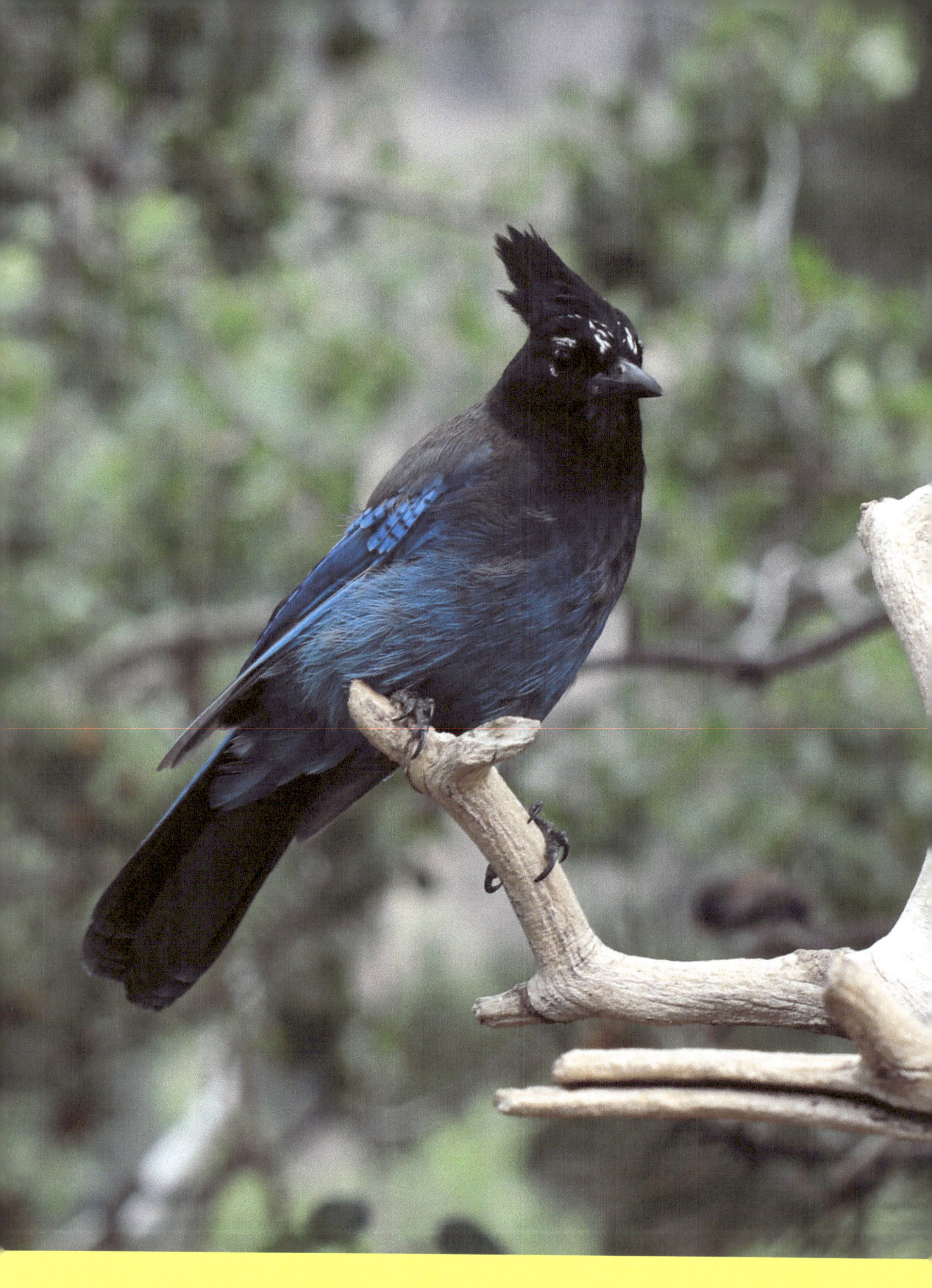

Stellar Jay

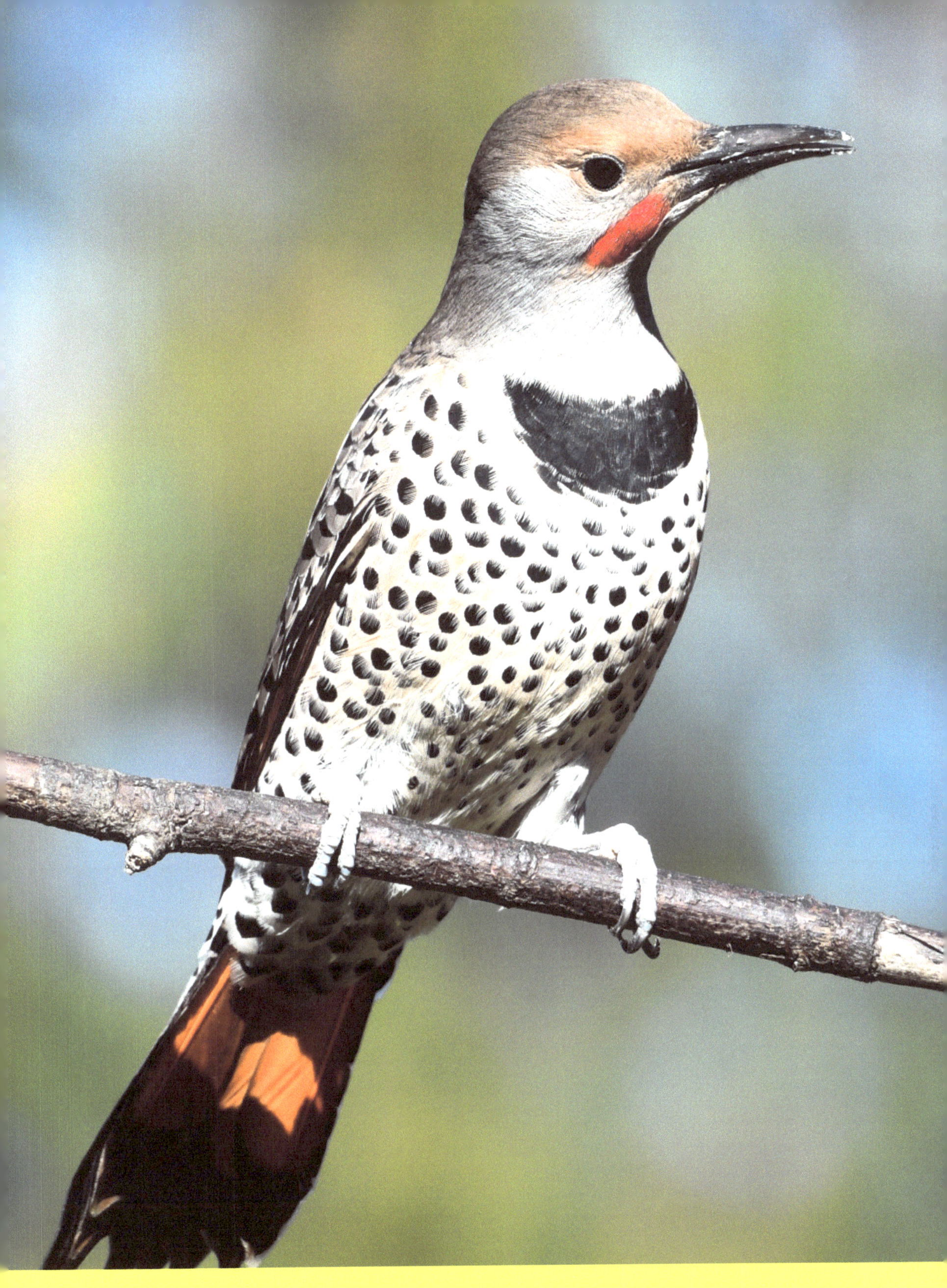

Northern Flicker

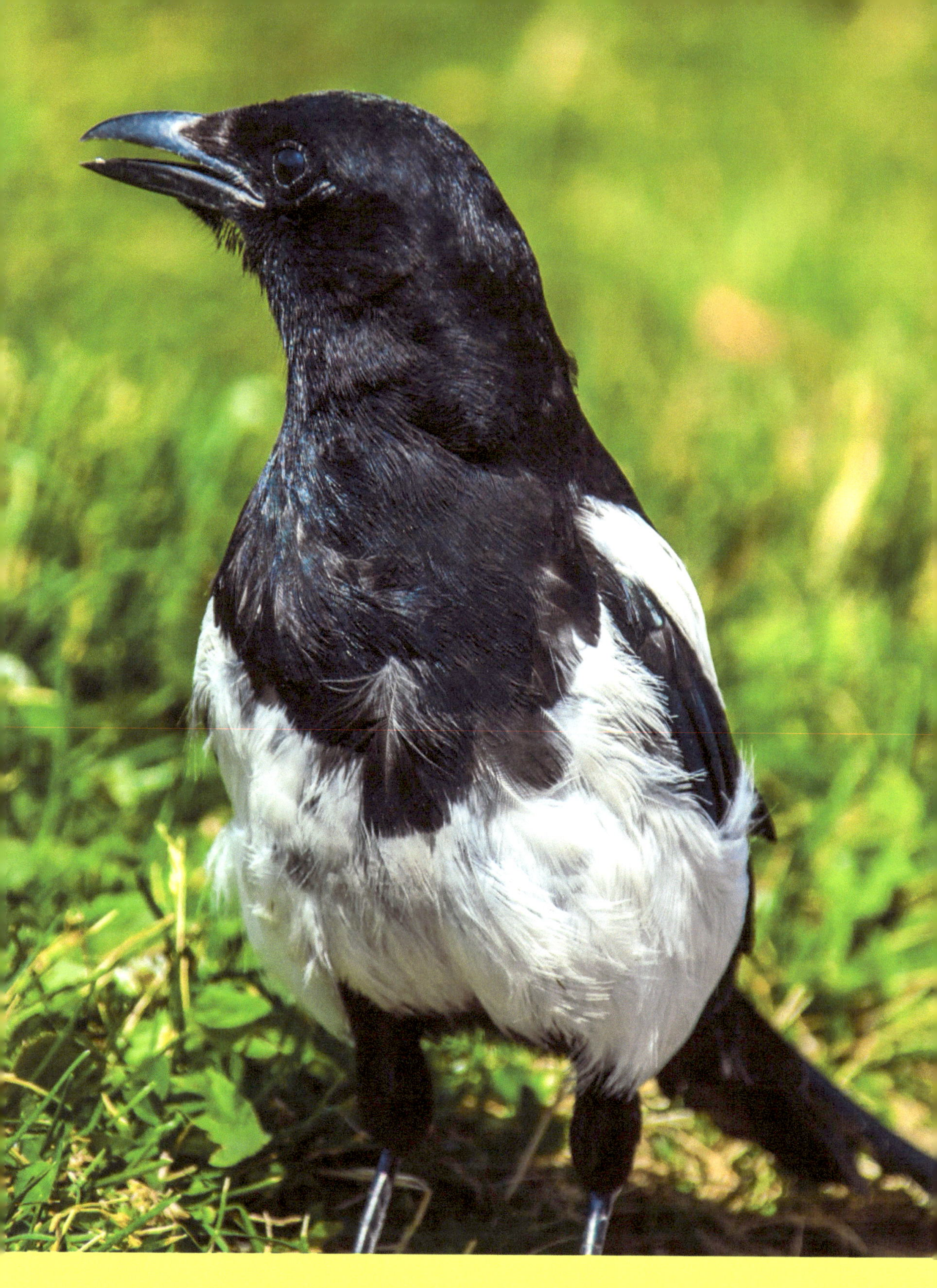

Black-billed Magpie

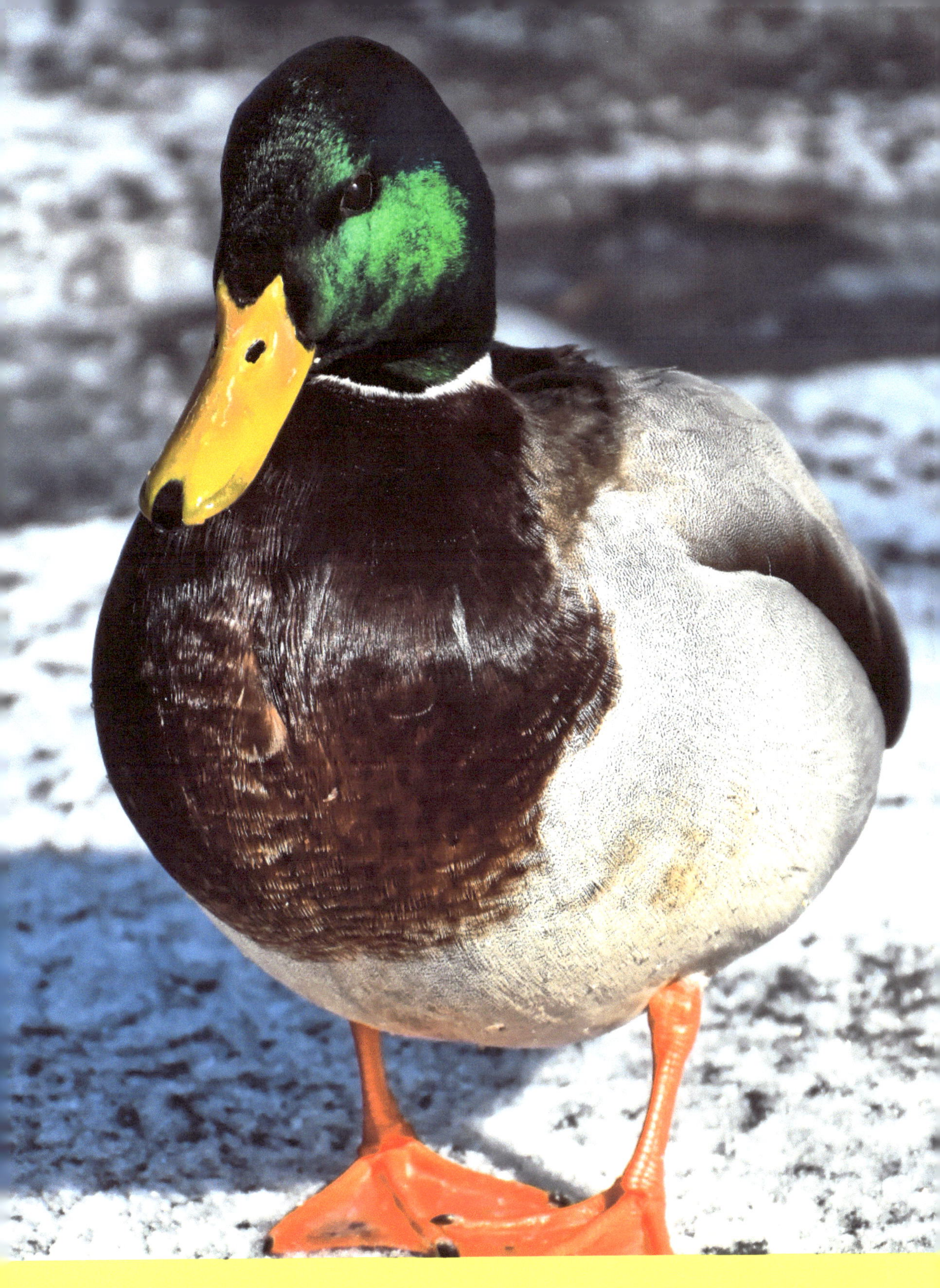

Mallard

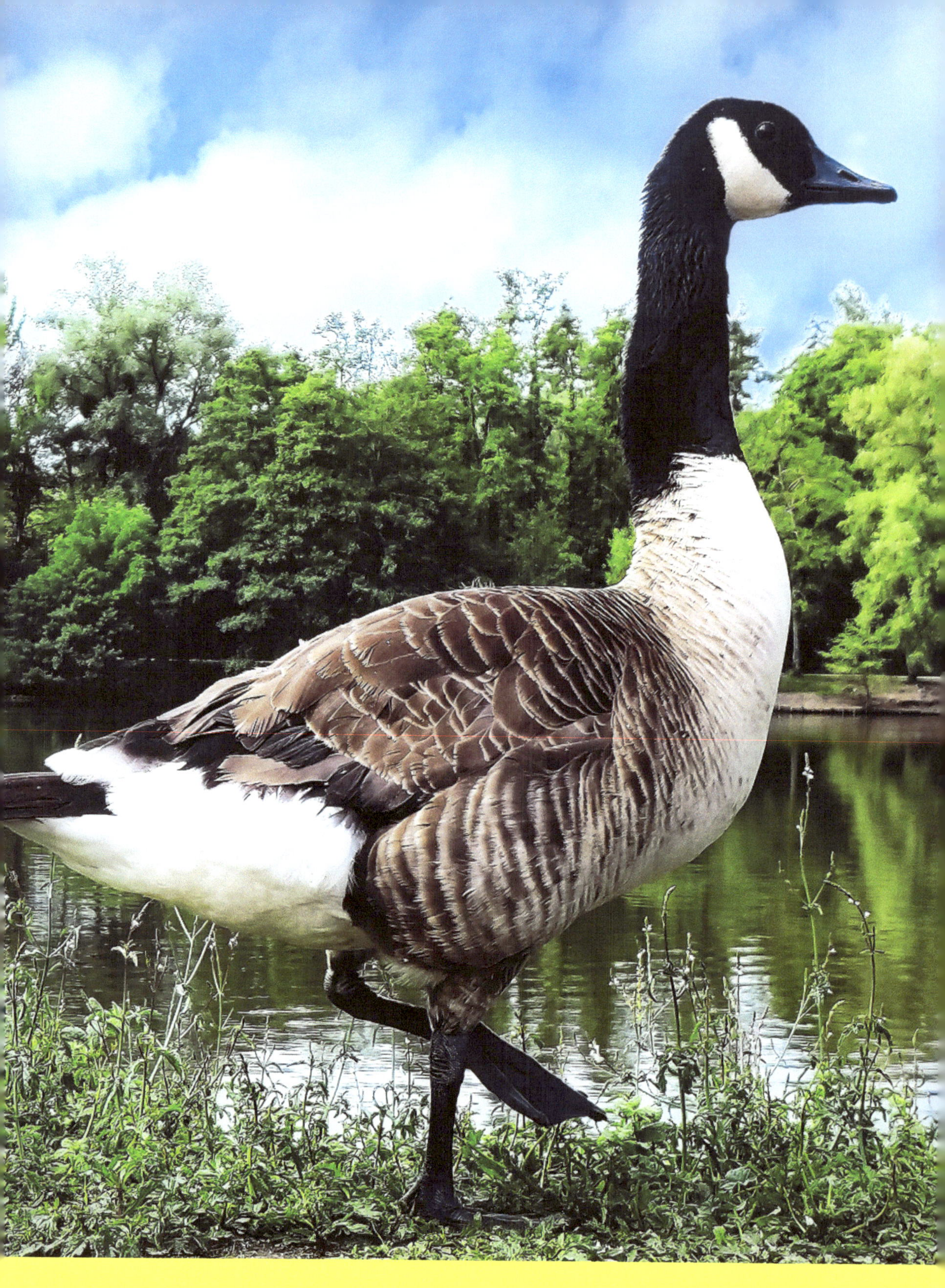

Canada Goose

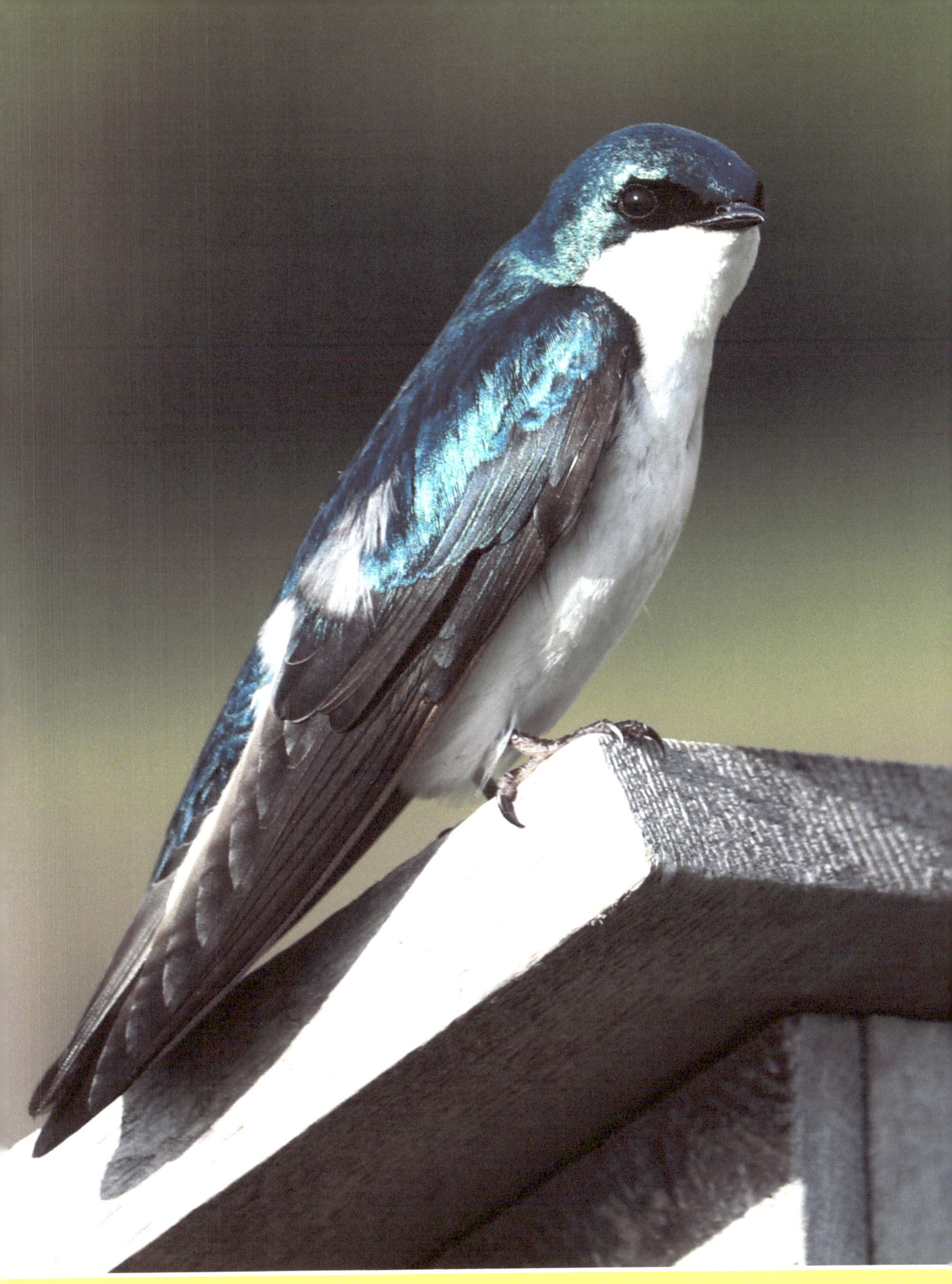

Tree Swallow

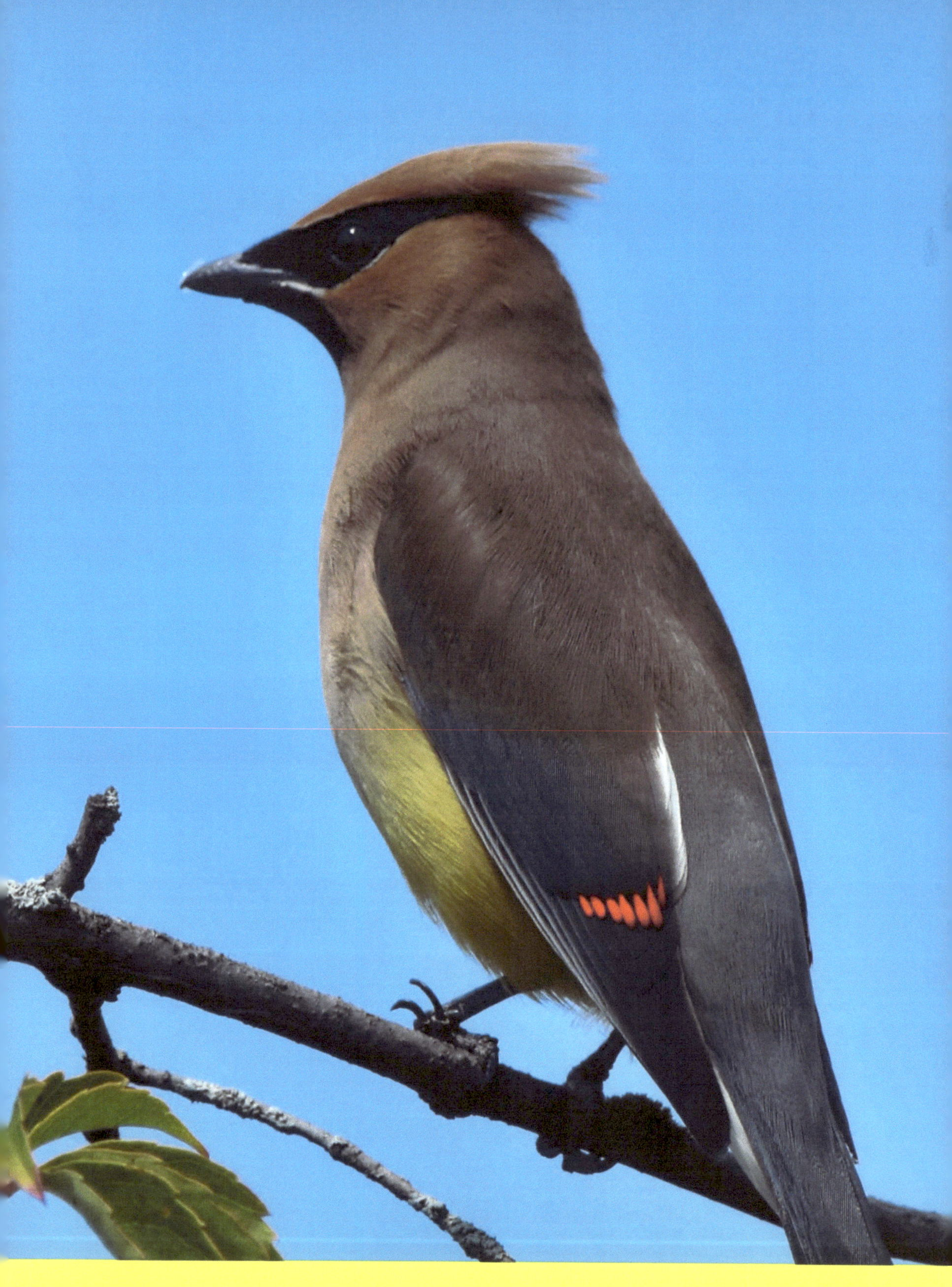

Cedar Waxwing

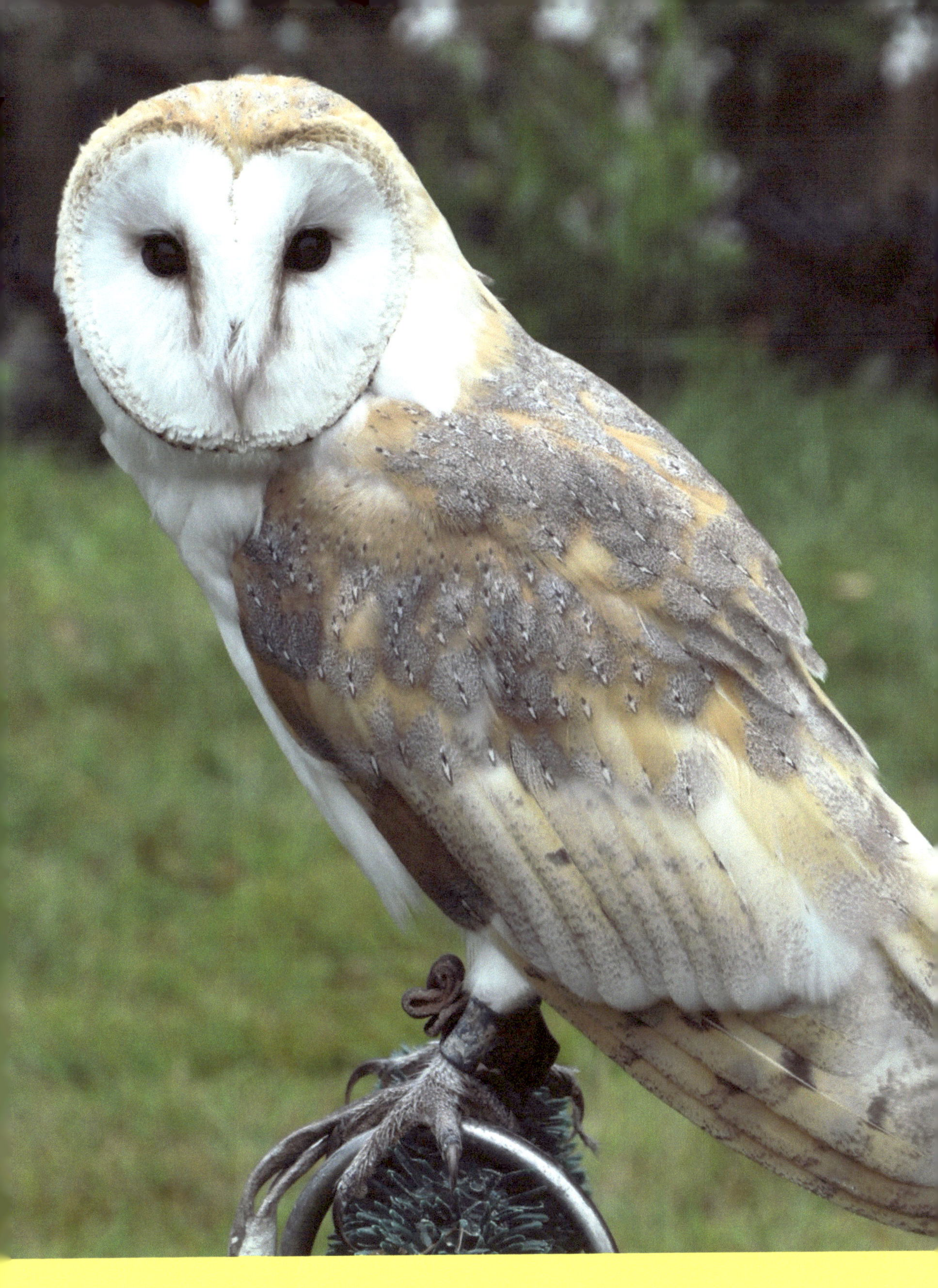

Barn Owl

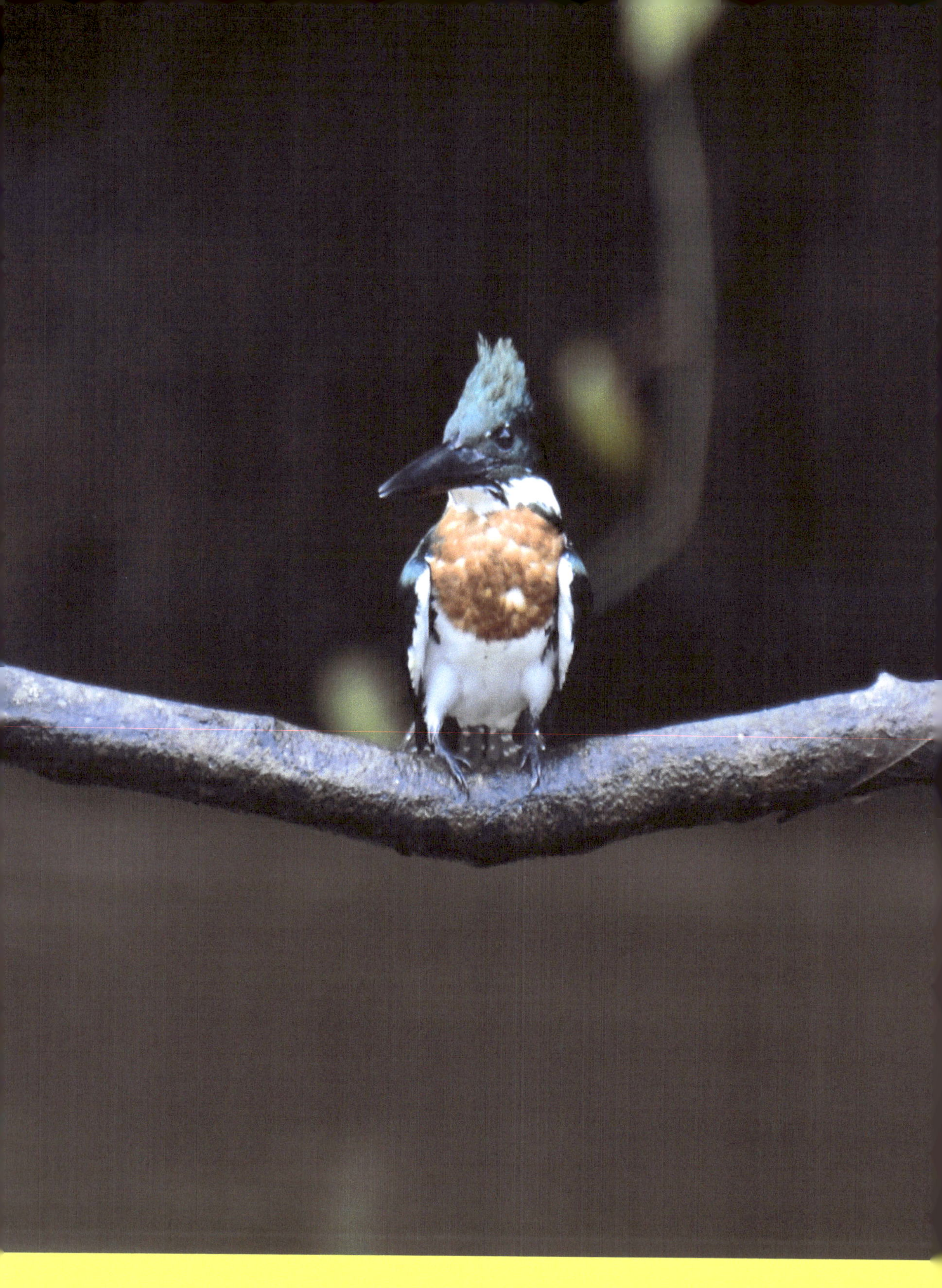

Belted Kingfisher

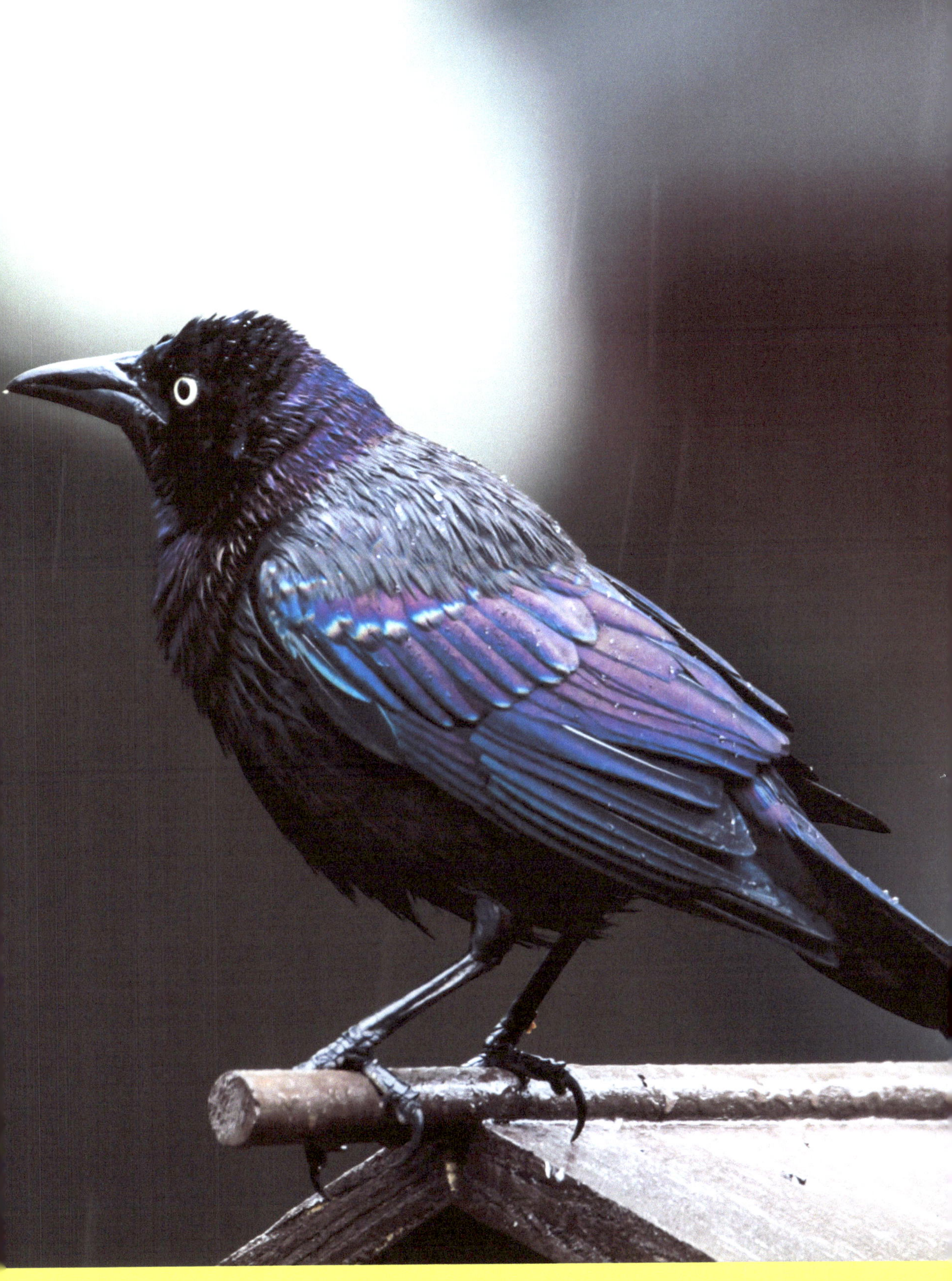

Grackle

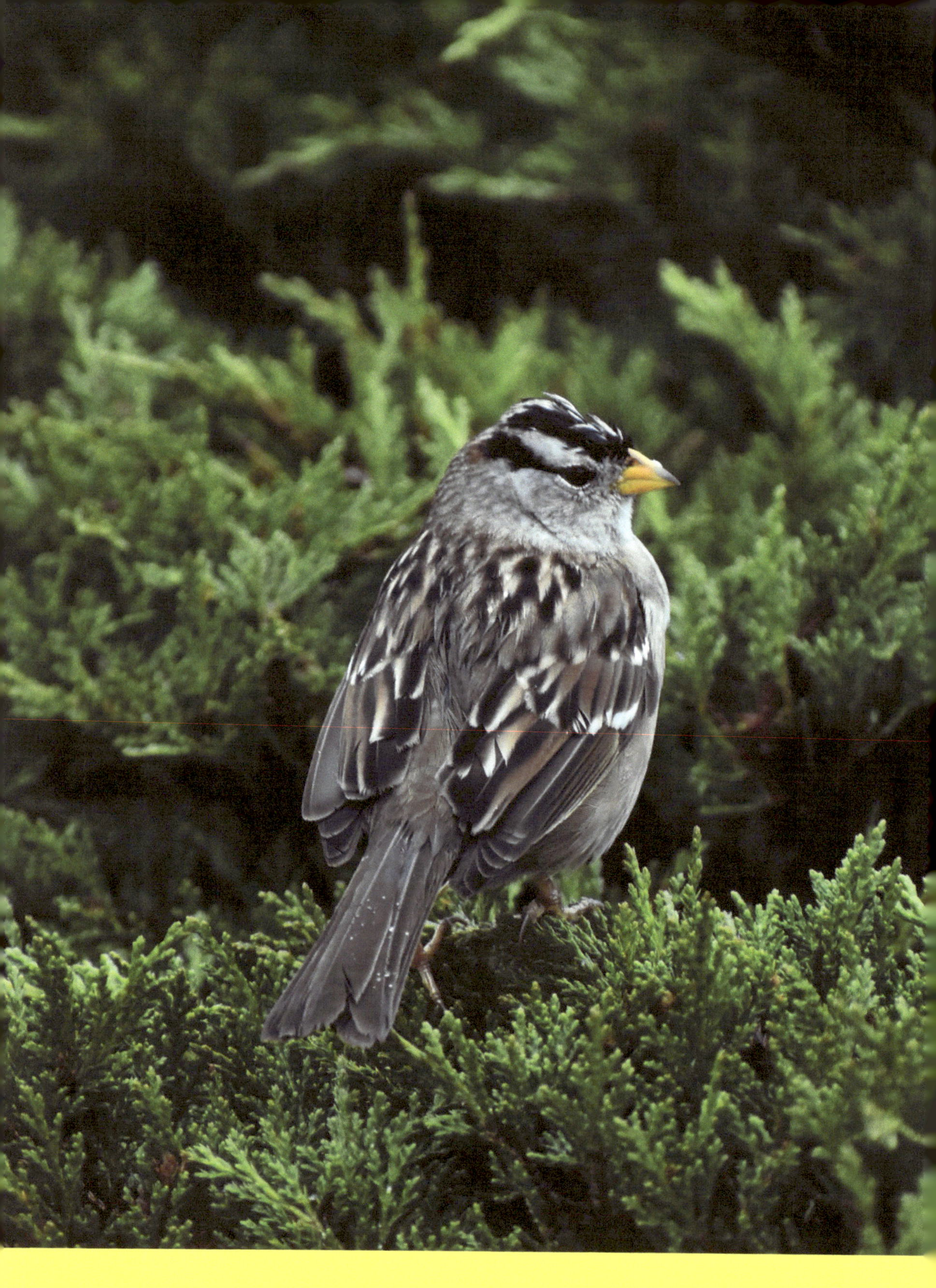

White Crowned Sparrow

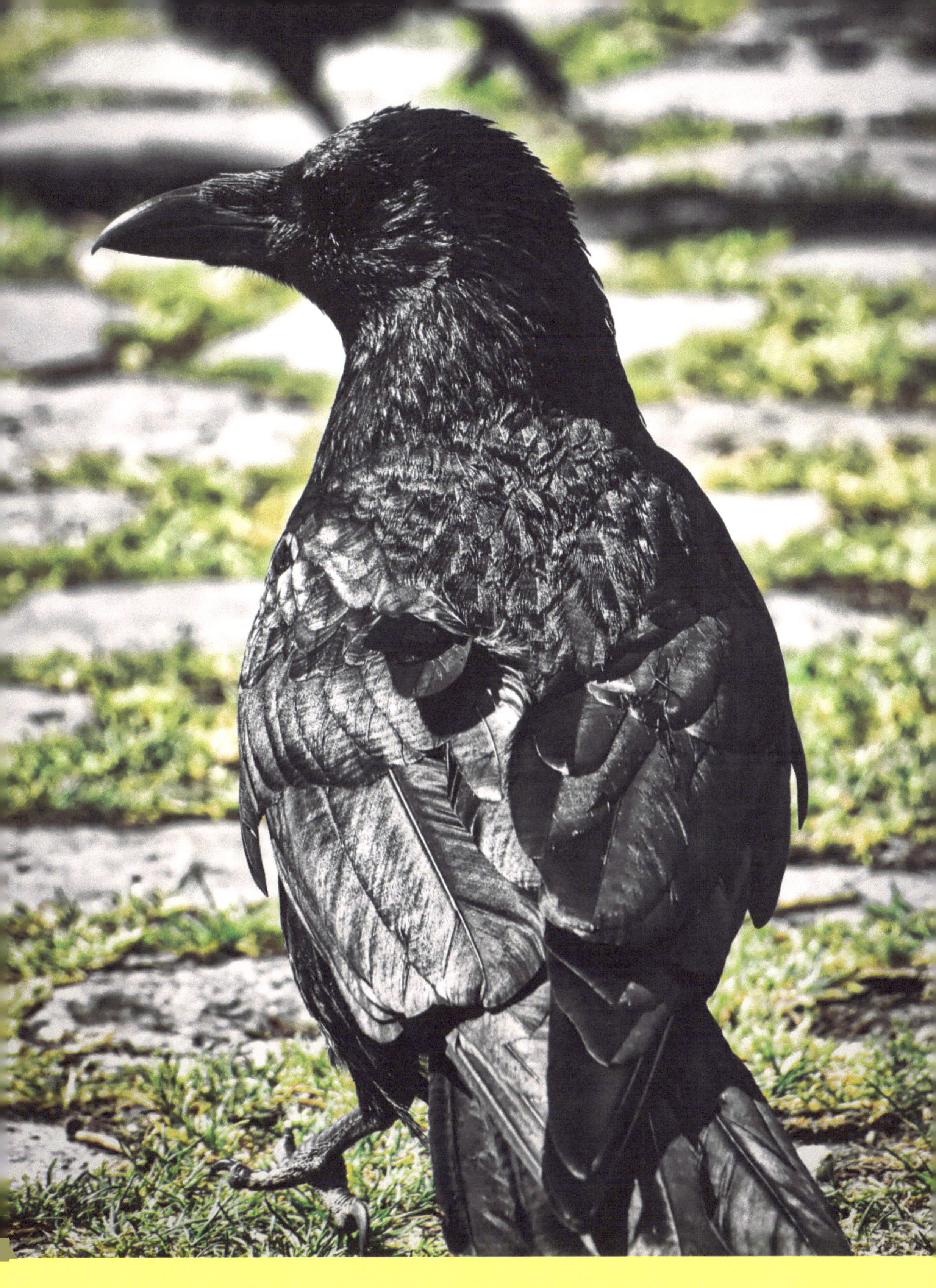

Common Raven

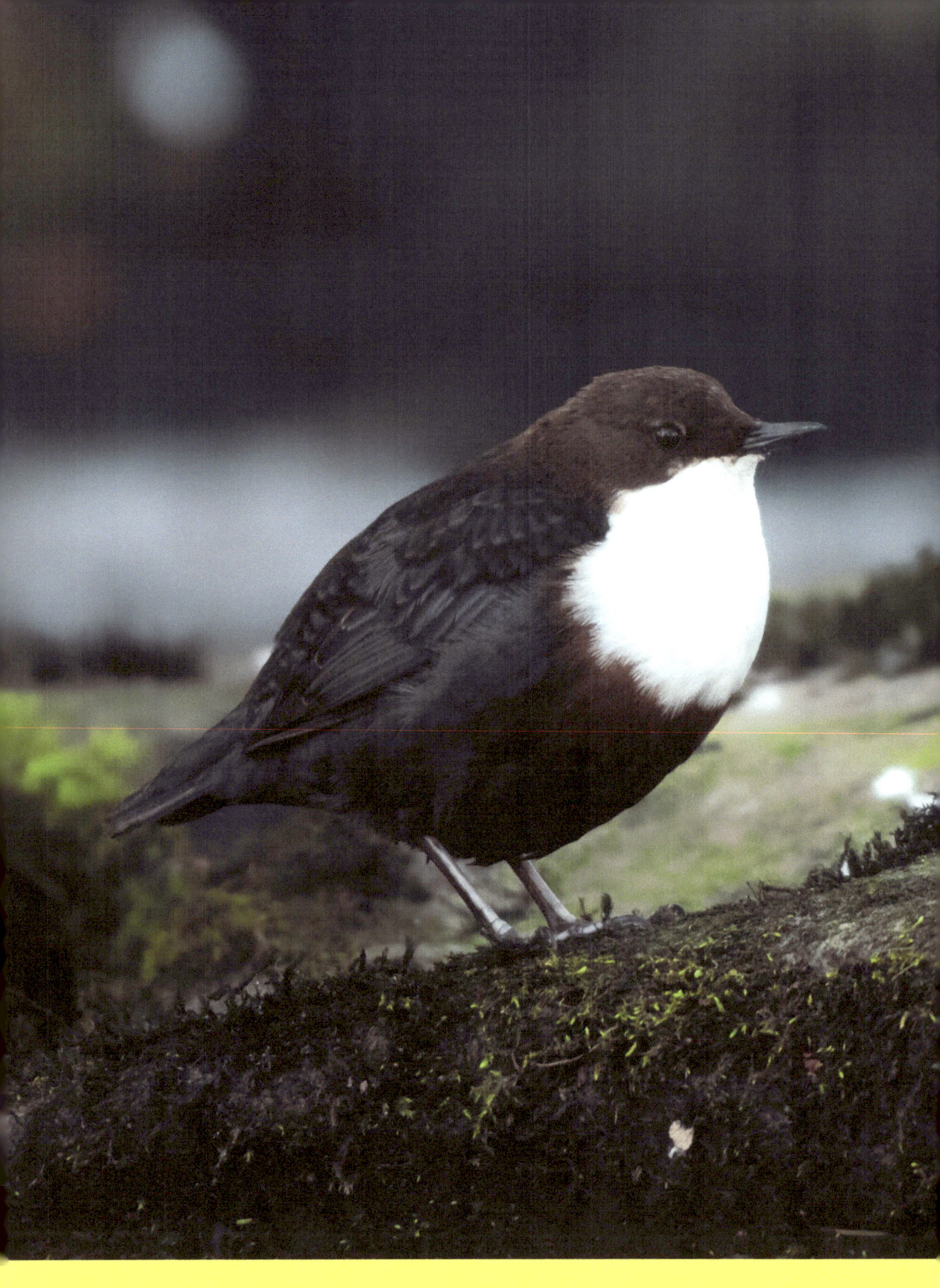

Dipper

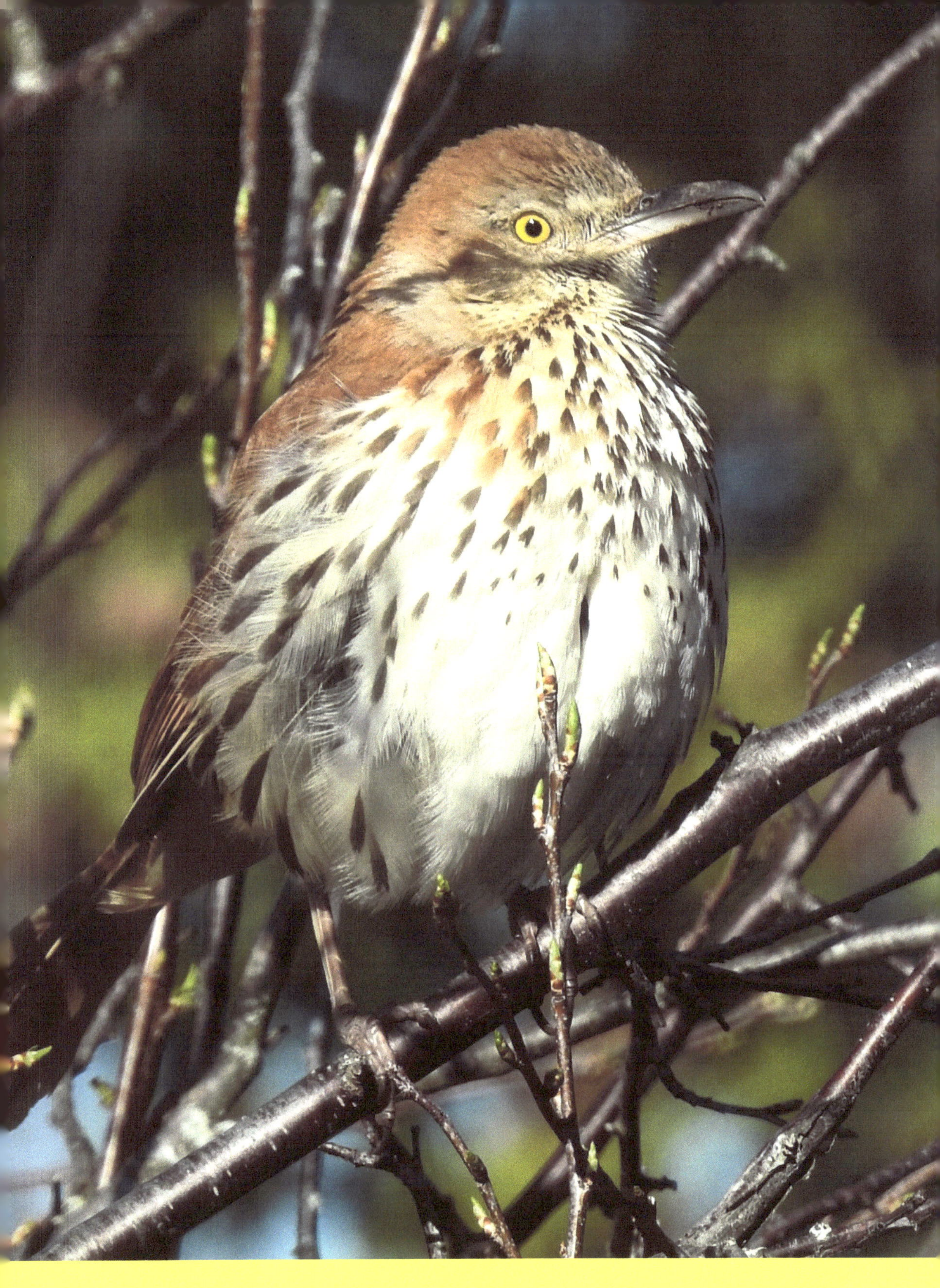

Brown Thrasher

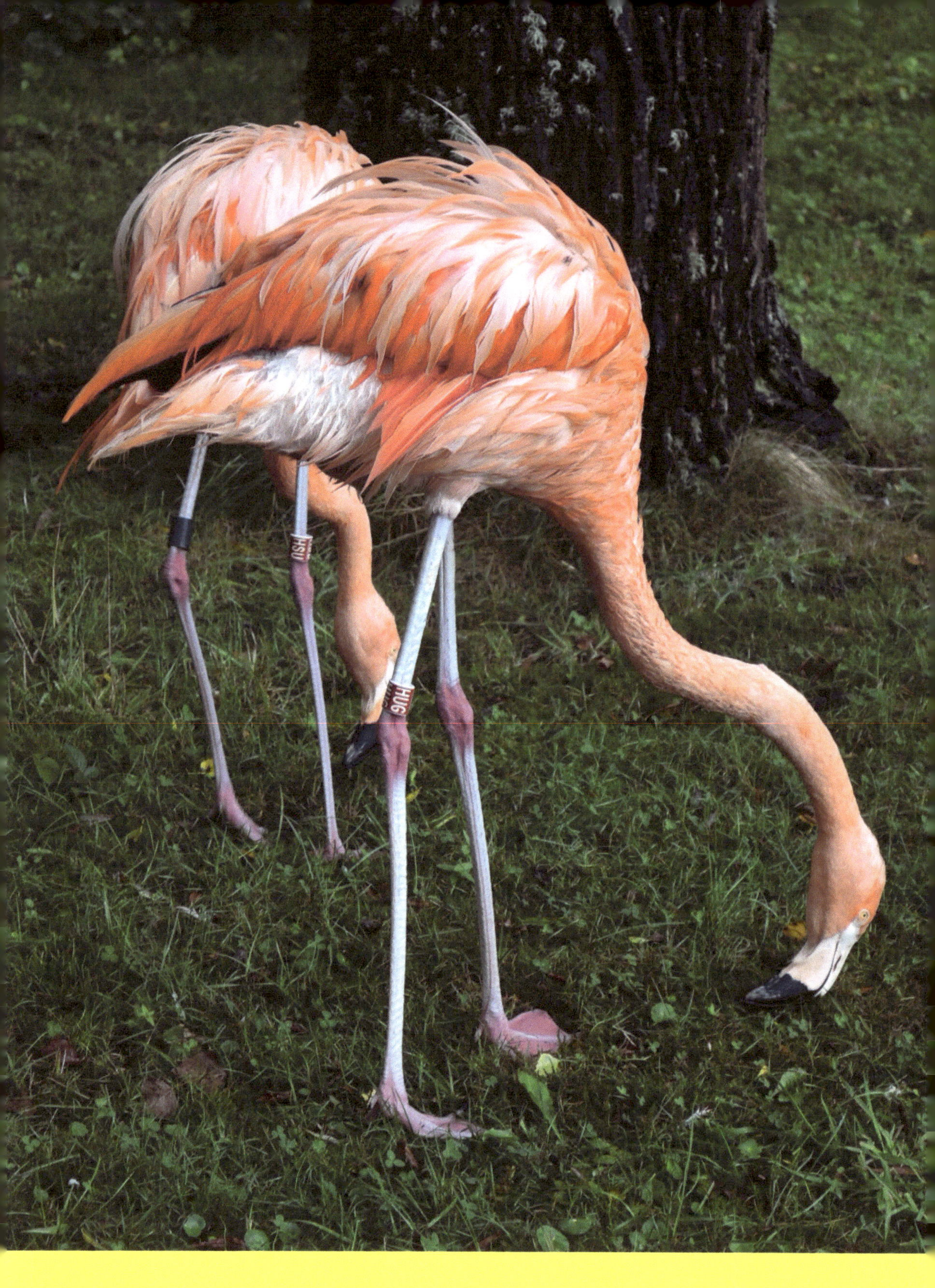

American Flamingo

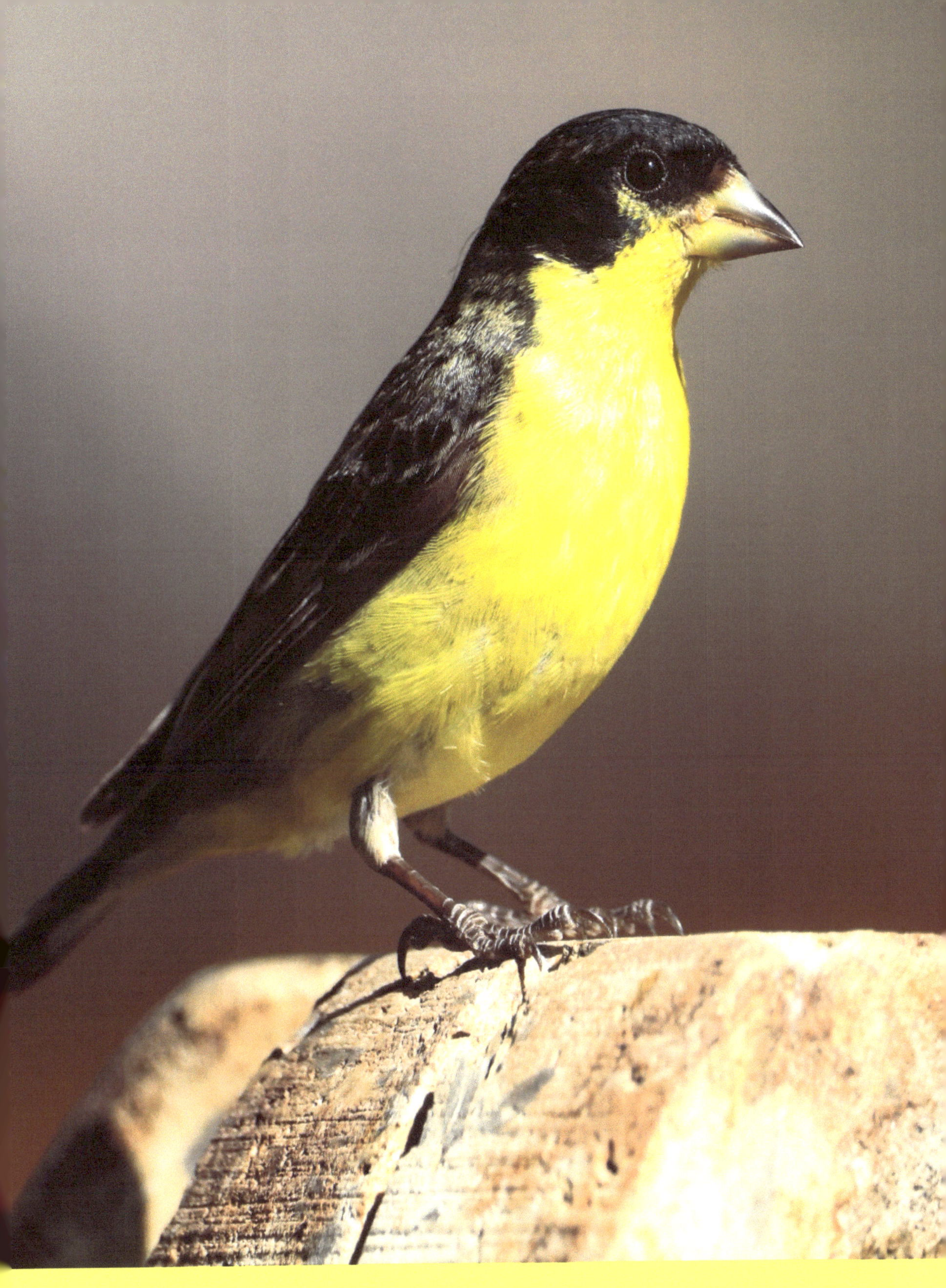

Lesser Goldfinch

www.ingramcontent.com/pod-product-compliance
Ingram Content Group UK Ltd.
Pitfield, Milton Keynes, MK11 3LW, UK
UKHW060116300726
14090UKWH00002B/228